D1783681

WORKING WOMEN
Your Guide to Coping with Pregnancy and Motherhood

WORKING WOMEN
Your Guide to Coping with Pregnancy and Motherhood

VERONICA CANNING

THE INDUSTRIAL SOCIETY

First published in 1997 by
The Industrial Society
Robert Hyde House
48 Bryanston Square
London W1H 7LN

© The Industrial Society 1997

ISBN 1 85835 457 9

British Library Cataloguing-in-Publication Data.
A catalogue record for this book is available from the
British Library

All rights reserved. No part of this publication may be
reproduced, stored in a retrieval system or transmitted, in
any form or by any means, electronic, mechanical,
photocopying, recording and/or otherwise without the
prior written permission of the publishers. This book may
not be lent, resold, hired out or otherwise disposed of by
way of trade in any form, binding or cover other than that
in which it is published, without prior consent of the
publishers.

Typeset by: GCS
Printed by: The Lavenham Press Ltd
Cover by: Form Graphic Design

Cartoons: John Byrne

The Industrial Society is a Registered Charity No. 290003

This book is dedicated to
Amber, Christopher and Peter

Acknowledgements
I would like to thank my husband Peter and daughter Amber for their incredible help and support for the working mother in their life. Without Christopher there would be no book as his arrival provided the inspiration for this project and much joy to our family.

I would also like to thank my colleagues Pamela Donnelly and John Byrne for their wonderful support and encouragement in the writing of this book.

CONTENTS

introduction

If you're reading this you're probably planning to be pregnant, are pregnant, or are about to become a working mother. If so, good luck. I know what it's like. I've worked in a variety of roles starting at the bottom and also working at Chief Executive level. I have two children of my own, and also have lots of friends and colleagues who have had children while continuing to hold jobs.

Through my own experience I've seen the problems encountered by women when pregnant, particularly when they become working mothers. I and many of my friends have found it hard to find all the information we needed in one place. In writing this book I've set out to fill that gap and I hope this book will be your one stop resource guide.

My two children were born several years apart and I found combining work, pregnancy and motherhood the second time much easier. This was mainly because I availed of the information and applied the principles in this book. Other women who have applied the same methods have also reported significant improvements in their ability to cope.

Being pregnant, working through pregnancy, returning to work and facing up to the new dual role of mother and worker can be both exciting and frightening.

You are the same person you always were but your physical, emotional and psychological needs will change. This book deals with each separate phase.

Chapters 1 and 2 will help you reduce stress and

continue to work effectively during your pregnancy.

Even though every pregnancy is different there are basics which every woman should know. Foremost are your rights as a working pregnant woman. You need to be quite clear on these, so that you can get them. Chapter 3 is a good guide and will tell you about your time off, entitlements and financial benefits.

Chapter 4 will guide you through the difficult phase of returning to work after the baby. You will get help to decide whether to want to return to work full-time or to work in an alternative way. It will also help you plan to ease back into work over a number of weeks.

The last phase is your first year as a working mother and it is definitely the most challenging. If you survive that 12 months, you'll survive anything. In Chapter 5, you'll discover whether you are a "supermum" or not. You'll learn working mothers' most useful word: no and lots of other ways of coping with your new role.

Finding good childcare is fundamental to a successful return to work. After reading the section in the appendix you'll be able to tackle this challenge and choose a suitable arrangement for you and your family.

Finally let me wish you the very best in your dual role. Remember you're not alone. You're one of an increasing group of mothers who are choosing to stay in the workforce.

1 reducing stress during pregnancy

The key to a successful working pregnancy is anticipating and preparing well for what will happen to you in your work day. This chapter will help you with this.

You may be lucky and sail through pregnancy with no problems at all but the reality for many is different. You can be nauseous and totally exhausted for the first three months, huge and out of breath for the last three months, and stressed by cramming a year's work into nine months so none of your workmates will say you went on a "holiday" for three months.

To pull off the miracle of a pregnancy that has minimum impact at work takes thought and preparation and a focus on using your time wisely.

To do your job well while pregnant means you must use your time more effectively than ever before — "time management" becomes crucial to your life.

A combination of thinking ahead, planning and managing your time will ensure that you reach the beginning of your maternity leave with all your work done, your co-workers happy and everything prepared for the arrival of your baby.

There are now some new factors operating in your life — you may try to ignore them but it's far better to include them in your preparation for working through pregnancy.

NEW FACTORS IN YOUR WORK LIFE DURING PREGNANCY

- Sickness.
- Telling your boss about your pregnancy/ dealing with the reactions of your co-workers.
- Taking time off for visits to doctor.
- Fatigue, carrying extra weight.
- Getting ready for hospital, buying supplies for your baby.
- Finishing up — feeling separation anxiety about leaving work.

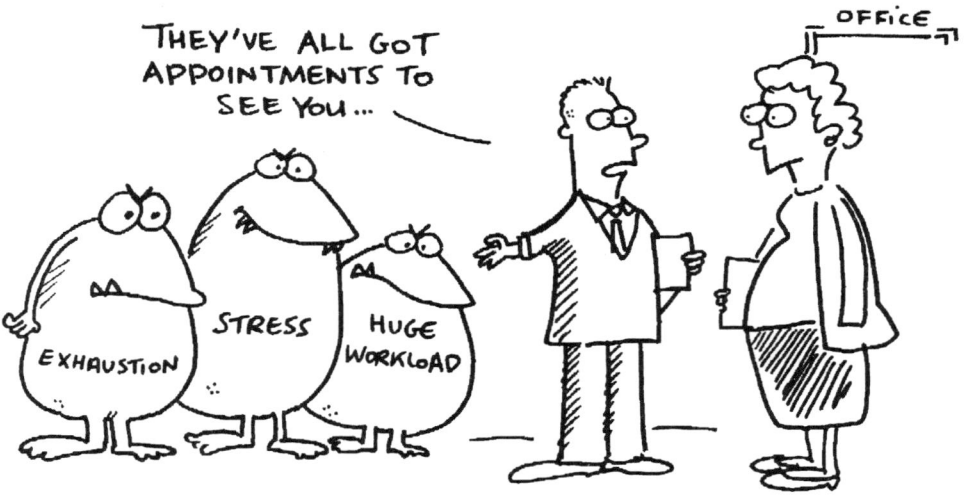

What is time management?

The concept of time management often frightens people — it shouldn't — managing your time is based on common sense. People unfamiliar with the concepts of time management often have misconceptions about it — I call these myths. Before we discuss how you manage your time let's debunk some of those myths.

THE COMMON MYTHS

When I'm pregnant I won't have enough time to do everything. You have the same amount of time as always. How you manage it is what's important.

I will have to pack in more things to save time. Time is perishable, you spend it not save it. It's not how much you do but what you do.

I must work longer hours now to make up for any slowness. Ever heard of diminishing returns?

I'll be more productive if I work harder than ever before. If you plan and know what you want to achieve you'll be in control without having to make extra efforts.

TIME MANAGEMENT MYTHS

Experience tells us everyone wastes time at work and in their personal lives. We blame others for time wasted, saying they interrupted us, stayed talking too long or kept us waiting. We also use lack of time to explain why we have not finished our work on time or let tasks pile up. As we cannot make more time, we have to achieve good results in the time we have. It's worth noting how many hours we have in each year as Debra Allcock's "Time and Workload Management" points out:

- There are 8760 hours available in the year
- 2920 spent sleeping
- 1928 spent at work
- 1664 hours available at weekends (not including sleeping)
- 320 hours of holiday (not including weekends) depending on our holiday allowance
- 1446 hours 'spare' during the working week (bearing in mind that actually it's really half of time i.e., 723, if you use the example above as a guideline)
- 482 hours travelling.

GUIDING PRINCIPLES OF USING YOUR TIME WISELY

There are three principles which you should learn before we discuss the actual practice of time management.

1. Pareto Principle

Now that time is so precious it's important to learn about the Pareto Principle. Simply put, it says that 80% of your productivity will come from 20% of your effort. In other words, don't confuse activity with accomplishment. It is important to do the 20% that yields the 80%, especially when time is precious during pregnancy and maternity leave.

2. The Apple Pie Approach To Life

When faced with a big pie you cut it up into many little slices in order to eat it. Visualise a report or stock-take that has to be done and you need a week to do it. Who has a week to devote to one job? No one. But everyone has an hour every day. Make a list of all the steps needed and do one every day. Don't try to swallow the whole thing at once. When faced with a large job it really does work — remember that.

3. The Orange And Grape Approach

Imagine each important A task is an orange and each C task is a grape. You clear the bowl of oranges — you're left with all the little grapes that fell between the bigger oranges. By themselves they are insignificant but a whole bowl of them mounts up — they are your less important tasks — your C tasks. Do them when you have 5 or 10 minutes to spare. For example, while waiting to meet someone, while holding on the phone, while sitting in a doctor's waiting room. List C tasks and concentrate on getting rid of them over time. They can clutter your mind.

Remember: beware the difference between urgent and important.

An undone C task can become urgent if left undone but it could still be unimportant in the grand scale of things.

TIME MANAGEMENT IN ACTION

1. Make Lists

Comprehensive List
Introduce to-do lists into your life. There are different kinds but you'll find that an overall list of everything is a good start. List all your tasks and assign each a priority, A, B or C and a date by which they must be done. Remember to include visits to doctor, taking rest and exercise, shopping for baby, telling your boss about your pregnancy. You don't have to necessarily work in an office to do this; shop assistants, librarians, schools teachers can all make lists of their tasks.

Daily To-Do List
Extract from your overall list the personal and work tasks you're going to do tomorrow. Take a page and divide it into two halves, work and personal. Fill in your tasks in order of priority eg. putting all your A tasks first.

2. Prioritise

Remember to put the priority beside each item. You only have to do one or two of your A tasks to get that 80% pay off. Doing 15 C tasks may make you feel you are busy but it won't give you the same pay off. If you have to write a report, do a stock-take or correct homework give it its correct priority.

3. Allocate Time To Each Task

A list of tasks is no use if you don't allocate time to each one. It's amazing how you find you overestimate what you'll achieve when you make lists each evening. After a few days of giving each task a time you become more realistic about how long everything takes and how to speed up. In some jobs you may find it more difficult to allocate specific time to tasks — especially if you are looking after customers, as in a shop or restaurant. Remember, try to pace yourself.

4. Reward Yourself

No matter what work you do it is important to pat yourself on the back and say well done — this week you've done all your A tasks and you should go home at the weekend feeling good. Buy that scarf you've been admiring — you can't buy belts or gorgeous skirts anymore. It's amazing how many neck adornments pregnant women have — it's the only place that doesn't swell.

5. End Each Day With The Plan For The Next Day — Your Secret Weapon.

At the end of each day take 15 minutes to take stock of the day and review your tasks and see how you've done. Concentrate on your A tasks but don't forget the B and C tasks. See how your energy levels were and are you being realistic in what you are asking yourself to do. Make your list for the next day and allocate time to each task. Remember when you come in the next morning, you'll know exactly what to do first.

Barti Patel, a radio producer with a local radio station in a large city, found the nature of her job required contacting large numbers of people at all hours of the day. They were often out or promised to call back, and it was getting increasingly difficult to keep track of how much progress she was actually making. She started using lists and working her way through them. She found that by writing out her list of possible contacts at the end of the day, she knew exactly where to start when she came in the next day. She did this each day for each of her radio programmes and found her stress levels reduced because she was always on top and able to update everyone on progress on a daily basis.

SEPARATE LISTS FOR YOUR PREGNANCY

Freeing your mind to concentrate on your work during work time is important. To minimise distractions caused by worrying about things like baby clothes and if you have got everything for the hospital, you should make your lists and plans for pregnancy separately.

Being ready to go to the hospital is probably the biggest worry — you might get caught napping with no appropriate clothes ready.

Make lists — get a notebook to keep in your handbag so you can write things down as you think of them.

- Hospital list for you
- Hospital list for baby
- List of baby's needs in first few weeks at home

Try to maximise your energy by shopping intelligently, use catalogues, phone up in advance to see if supplies are available.

KNOW YOUR BEST WORK TIME

No one, especially a pregnant woman, can possibly keep going at the same speed and efficiency all day. Every woman has her own peaks and valleys. Find out yours. Be most productive at your times of highest energy. Find out your best times by filling in this chart over 3 work days.

Time	Low	Medium	High
8am			
9am			
10am			
11am			
12am			
1pm			
2pm			
3pm			
4pm			
5pm			
6pm			
7pm			
8pm			
9pm			

Usually people are at their highest energy levels in mid-morning but remember pregnancy can knock your usual rhythm out — especially if you are feeling sick. When you discover the two to three hour block in the day when you are at your best, use it wisely. Only do A tasks and things that are demanding. Be vigilant about keeping this peak time for yourself and your priorities. Many jobs, like shop work, have their own inbuilt time constraints but if you know your best and worst times you could try to change your shift accordingly.

If you work in an office try to discourage interruptions — either in person or by phone. Remember you're working to a deadline — 9 months — and you want to make sure all the important things you're responsible for are done before you leave. This may not be possible if you work for someone else and need to respond to their demands.

*For **Helen Johnson**, a senior manager in an insurance company, discovering that her best time was 11.00am — 1.30 meant that she kept all her major work — A tasks — until that time. She arranged with her secretary not to be disturbed and she worked away, often having a light sandwich at her desk. She took a later lunch and spent the afternoon on the phone and in meetings. She went home every evening happy that she was getting some of her A tasks done every day. This was particularly useful as it came to the end of her pregnancy and she knew she had to finish a number of important jobs before she left for maternity leave.*

A handy hint is to do the most difficult thing first when you get to work. The rest of the day will flow more smoothly when that worry is out of the way. When pregnant you tend to lose concentration and get more tired as the day goes on — completing a task early in the day that could become a worry if undone, is good time management and reduces stress greatly.

TIME OFF FOR CHECK UPS

It is vital that you schedule in your visits for your check ups.

5 TIPS TO MINIMISE DISRUPTION AT WORK

- **If possible choose a place near your work, to reduce travel time and stress.**
- **Try and have appointments at the beginning or end of the day** as you can then go to work and stay there — if you leave at 11am or 3pm you're obviously missing.
- **Don't schedule an important meeting or visit out of your work place immediately after the appointment.** Remember you could be delayed. You could be sitting in the waiting room when some other woman might decide to deliver and need the doctor more.
- **Do some C tasks.** Bring some work-related reading or use the time to make lists, especially ones which are related to the pregnancy — that way you get to check your lists and your progress in completing tasks on a regular basis.
- To avoid coming back to work frustrated **bring a list of questions** with you so that all your queries are answered.

How can you relax at work?

Your extra weight and the fatigue of the first and third trimester really slow you down. Trying to ignore the difference in your physical self can cause stress — in addition to all the normal causes of stress in every job. The key is learn to relax so that you can appear to be doing the same job you've always done. Easier said than done you say, my work would not allow me to take time out. This is certainly true of some jobs but remember every job allows you some breaks, including lunch each day — use these times for your relaxation.

TAKE TIME AND SET THE SCENE FOR RELAXATION

- Find a private spot at work
- Make it comfortable
- Make this a priority - remove things that distract you.
- Set aside time every day, best if it is a lunch time — the same so that you build up a habit. Habits take time to form — usually constant repetition every day for a month establishes a habit — so persevere.

If your job does not allow you to take time out at all — do this immediately you get home before you face into the evening's activities.

READY, STEADY, RELAX — THE THREE STEPS

1. Breathe

It's amazing how you catch your breath, even hold your breath, when you're stressed — especially in the third trimester when your lungs are squashed. Slowly breathe in through your nose and out through pursed lips — count to five on the way out. Keep breathing nice and light — don't pant.

2. Unknot the muscles

The secret is to tighten a muscle and then relax it. Then you really realise what a relaxed muscle is. Often you tense up muscles unknowingly. Start with arms, and move out to legs, feet and end with face — tense each muscle and then relax.

3. De-stress the mind

You want to give the over-active mind a break — you're trying to organise work, your home to get ready for the baby. Build in a time out period every day. Relax all your muscles and breathe normally. Choose a word and repeat it to yourself saying it in time with your breathing. Try to concentrate on the word — forget all your problems — it's only 10 minutes — nothing will self-destruct if you switch off.

EIGHT TIPS FOR REDUCING STRESS IN WORK

1. Try to get as much rest and sleep as possible.
It's easy to say but with an active bump and an even more active bladder it's difficult. Remember you don't have to be asleep to rest — just be in bed with your feet up.

2. Immediately eliminate major causes of stress.
Don't move house, change jobs, volunteer to start a fund-raising venture for your club. Keep on an even keel.

3. Organise, organise, organise and eliminate minor causes of stress. Work your brain not your body — have a plan of what you want to do and do things one at a time.

4. Don't take on other people's burdens — watch out for the monkeys. Think of tasks as monkeys. Every time someone comes into the room with a family of monkeys on their back and tries to give them to you — refuse; make sure they leave complete with the whole family — don't accept even one extra task that's not yours.

5. Exercise: walk it off. Telling a pregnant woman to exercise is daft — you probably think being pregnant is exercise enough. However, walking or a spot of tidying will get your mind off stress, especially useful when the nesting instinct takes over and you tidy anything that's stationary — even things that have been there for years get tidied.

6. Talk to people. Now is the time to unburden yourself to friends and family. After all they've been doing this to you for years — you'll feel much better

11

when you realise how many other women feel like you. A word of caution — don't do this with work colleagues.

7. You can't change the world — at least not in this nine months period. Accept that some problems at work are not going to be solved before you go on maternity leave. Don't exhaust yourself. Use your energies to do things you can finish before maternity leave.

8. Remember to have fun. Remember to build into every week some fun time — you'll relax, switch off and be all the better in work for it. Fun lunches once a week, a visit to the cinema or theatre. Do it now — it won't be so easy when you have a baby.

Jane Sykes works as a receptionist in a large advertising agency. Luckily she was sitting all day but even with that she found she was getting very stiff and uncomfortable especially in the last trimester. She used her morning and afternoon breaks to do the ready, steady, relax — three steps. She found it helped her greatly. Her employer made a small room available to female staff and so she had no problems there.

Can you be comfortable in work?

Almost every pregnant woman feels some discomforts in work at some stage in her pregnancy. They are mainly a cause of irritation rather than fright and this section gives some suggestions to reduce their effects. However, it is important to remember that in exceptional cases women have to take time off due to complications of pregnancy like pre-eclampsia. They should be treated like any other illness and usual leave should apply.

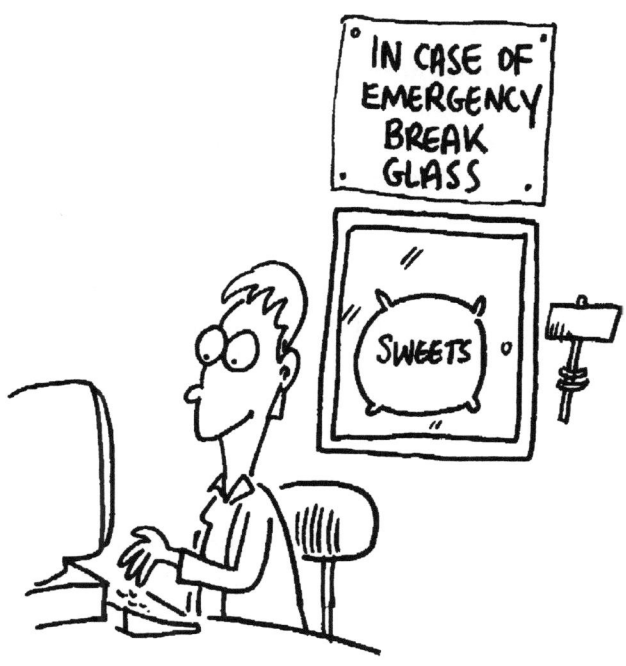

HOW TO LOOK LIKE YOU'RE DOING THE JOB — WHILE HAVING MORNING SICKNESS.

The first thing to realise is that it must have been a man who coined the term "morning sickness". It can, if you're unlucky, be all day, any time sickness.

- Have an escape hatch ready — always sit near the door at meetings.
- If you're going to be sick or pass out you should get out ar_ deal with it outside. Don't draw attention to yourself and distract your co-workers.
- If you're speaking or giving a class — take a break.
- Keep a pregnancy survival pack (details at the end of the chapter) in your locker or desk.

HEALTH PROBLEMS — WORK FROM HOME

If at any stage your physical discomfort is such that staying at work is not on, you may have to remain at home. If you have a job where the work or output is what matters — not your actual presence — then you could

Discomforts	Solutions
Nausea & getting sick Especially in trimester when you've not yet announced your pregnancy.	• Eat lightly & frequently, keep supplies at your work station. • Avoid heavy work lunches with co-workers. • Stay out of the canteen if it has strong smells. • Ask people not to smoke near you.
Fatigue Common in the first and end of third trimester	• Learn your body's rhythm and when you have more energy — do the most work then. • Take a rest and time out in the middle of the day, preferably during your lunch break – it'll get you through till quitting time. • Delegate – swop with co-workers. • Reduce worry – concentrate on important tasks. • Go to bed early.
Backache Especially as the bump grows	• When seated, raise your feet on a waste paper bin, or stack of files. If your job requires you to stand keep a high stool handy. • Never wear high heels – banish them. • Avoid lifting heavy objects. • Control weight gain.
Headaches common in pregnancy	• Rest, relax in a darkened room if possible. • Go for a walk in fresh air. • Reduce work place stress. • Use cold face cloths on face.

Discomforts	Solutions
Heartburn When stomach acid comes back into throat.	• Avoid certain foods, especially fatty foods so loved in canteens. Take a proper lunch break and eat little and often in day. • Drink water. • Ask doctor about antacids.
Overheating Pregnancy speeds up your metabolism	• Wear layers to work and you can peel on and off as you want. • Use survival bag to freshen up frequently. • Use a fan. • A small towel or hankies are useful to wipe hands.
Swelling Your kidneys are collecting more water than usual & it collects in your feet and hands.	• Keep your feet raised while sitting. Lie on your side during your day off if possible. • Pamper yourself by soaking your feet when you get home. • Wear loose clothes.
Breathlessness At the end of pregnancy when baby is pressing against diaphragm.	• Sit and stand straight to give your lungs as much room as possible. • Avoid rushing about and try to reduce going upstairs.

discuss working from home with your boss. Nowadays many successful businesses are run with a mobile phone, internet and a fax. Agree the body of work to be done and the deadline and work away. You can fax most things or use a courier service. It certainly demonstrates commitment to your boss and reduces stress as you feel things are not piling up waiting for your return.

HOW TO REDUCE EFFECTS OF MINOR DISCOMFORTS ON YOUR WORK

A bewildering array of things happen to your body but you'll find these tips cover the most common. There are many other changes in your body and if you are worried keep a list in your handbag and query your doctor or gynaecologist about them at your next visit. A good tip is to get yourself a comprehensive book and make it your guide.

Sharon Baldwin works on the jewellery counter in a large department store, so she has to stay in a confined space and usually on her feet. She was exhausted each evening and so resolved to try and find a solution. She began by getting an ordinary chair but found she was too low down while sitting and looked like she was slacking off. She found the perfect solution by bringing in a high stool from home and putting it into a corner of her area, against the wall. She leaned on it rather than sitting down and found it took the weight off her feet significantly to get her through the "bad" days when she was feeling more exhausted.

PREGNANCY WORK SURVIVAL PACK
- Plain biscuits, glucose sweets, or packet of raisins to keep sugar levels up.
- Bottle of water or fruit juice.
- Your favourite food — however bizarre, it's a great comfort.
- Grocery plastic bags for that awful moment — you'll probably never use them once you know they are there.

- Box of tissues or wipes — scented wipes are a great reviver if you're feeling off.
- A face cloth — great for freshening up — toothbrush and toothpaste.
- A fan or battery-operated fan — especially useful if you work in a building where you can't readily stick your head out of the window for fresh air.
- Antacids for heartburn and indigestion.
- Vitamins or iron tablets or prescribed medicines.
- Change of blouse.
- Deodorant and perfume — a light fragrance.
- Comfortable shoes — if feet swell during the day. Don't get caught walking around in bare feet — it doesn't give a very good image.
- Your book on pregnancy — which explains all those odd symptoms like spots before your eyes and metallic taste.

2 working effectively during pregnancy

Knowing how to communicate effectively with people in work and knowing your rights regarding your health and safety will go a long way to making your time at work during pregnancy as effective as possible.

Announcing your pregnancy to your boss and co-workers and dealing with their reactions is crucial because it needs to be handled correctly or it can affect how well you get on at work during your pregnancy. This chapter will help you with this important step.

Knowing your personal rights as a woman, how to be assertive, and some idea of the art of negotiation will be important to you now. This chapter goes through each of these and will leave you in a very strong position for holding your own with any co-worker, whatever their reaction to you!

The explanation of your safety rights in this chapter will help you greatly in clarifying your rights for negotiation with your employer.

Use the Pregnancy Plan on page 37 to guide you.

How will you announce your pregnancy in work?

There's nothing like contemplating the realities of

announcing your pregnancy to your boss, or surveying your work routine from the view point of pregnancy, to focus the mind.

You have to announce your news and make working while pregnant a reality. To survive the next 7-8 months it's important to re-tune your negotiation and assertiveness skills and remind yourself of your basic rights.

In addition, you should look at the physical side of your work and see if it is going to cause any problems.

SEVEN TIPS FOR ANNOUNCING YOUR PREGNANCY IN WORK

1. **Tell your boss or supervisor first.**
   It makes you look bad if someone else breaks the news first and you risk starting your working pregnancy off on a bad footing.

2. **Pick your time carefully.**
   Meet your boss at a stress free time of the day. Ensure that you have your boss's total attention, so don't announce it on the way to meet someone or on the way out the door in the evening. A note of caution — don't automatically assume that a female boss or supervisor will be more supportive because of their gender.

   However a boss is more likely to be sympathetic if she or his partner has been through a similar experience.

3. **Speak in private.**
   Ask to speak in private and plan to minimise disruptions by asking that his/her secretary hold calls.

4. **Be professional and positive.**
   Announce your pregnancy, state you're happy about it and that you'll be continuing to work. Show

that you're assuming it is a business as usual approach.

5. Hold off your news until after the first trimester is over.

There are a number of reasons for this — principally the risk of miscarriage is lower after the first trimester. An additional benefit is that you are reducing the length of time you are "officially" pregnant in work and of course the length of time people have to worry about it. With luck, in work terms, it can be a "five or six month pregnancy". If you are about to have a salary review or awaiting a decision on promotion you should wait until that is complete.

6. Beware if you have morning sickness.

You may not be able to wait so long. Your co-workers will notice if you go green and rush out the door on a regular basis.

7. Don't discuss maternity leave yet.

Don't rush the fences — it is best to assume that you'll be welcome back but let the boss digest your news first. Go into details of your arrangements for maternity leave later.

Barti Patel, who works in an independent radio station, had to choose her time to announce her pregnancy very carefully. Unfortunately she suffered badly with morning sickness and was finding it increasingly difficult to hide this. Her boss, Amanda, was very preoccupied with getting a major series of shows done, complicated by some domestic problems of her own. Barti was becoming quite anxious to announce the news to Amanda before someone else told her. She waited until the most difficult section of the series was done and then asked to have a meeting with Amanda. She told her the news, told her she was staying on at work and would discuss her maternity leave later when things were a little less hectic.

Amanda responded very well and appreciated Barti's thoughtfulness in waiting until the major show was ready, and complimented her on her professional approach.

***Jane Sykes**, a receptionist in an advertising agency, was very well and completely unaffected by morning sickness. She did not announce her news until she was four months pregnant. She had no problems as her company had a personnel department which told her that when they had the dates of her maternity leave, they would recruit a temporary replacement.*

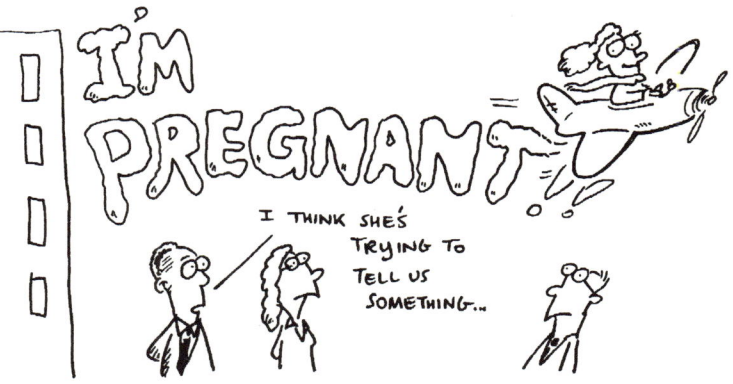

How will people react to your news?

Consider your co-workers' reactions to your announcement of pregnancy. You may be lucky and have a wave of solid warmth from all around you at work. However, you should be aware that not everyone at work may be as thrilled as you about your news. It's best to anticipate some mixed feelings and prepare for them. These feelings usually arise from people's own perceptions of what the pregnancy and maternity leave will mean to them.

- Some co-workers may be worried about having to carry your work load because they fear that you will not be able to do as much work as usual.

- Some co-workers may be resentful and think that you are trying to have it all by working and having a baby. They may feel that you should choose one role or the other and may resent your desire to both work and have a family.
- Some women co-workers may be feeling low as they may be trying to get pregnant and are having difficulty.
- It's hard to clearly interpret repeated attention to your physical condition. It could be genuine concern and support, but be careful — it could be that your boss or co-workers are concerned that you won't be able to do your job while pregnant or that you should give up work and prepare to have your child.
- It's important to be aware that people who have not had children may be less inclined to understand or may even be a little hostile.

UNDERSTANDING THE MOST COMMON MISCONCEPTIONS ABOUT WORKING PREGNANT WOMEN

A common worry for working mothers-to-be is how to maintain professionalism and assert their position as a worker in the new circumstances of their pregnancy.

It is a valid concern and it's important to understand other people's changed perceptions of you so that you can effectively deal with them.

There are a number of common misconceptions about pregnant women at work. They fall under three headings.

1. You are not going to be as committed to work now that you are pregnant.

You may be surprised to realise that some people can query your commitment to your job when you are pregnant, or that you can be taken less seriously as a worker.

It may be considered that your priorities have shifted away from work to home and family. If this doubt about your commitment and your performance exists it can be a real barrier to you in your work. Your boss's attitude may change, your co-workers' attitudes may change and if you're not fully aware of what is happening your attitude and performance will be adversely affected in turn.

To break out of this you have to clearly demonstrate your commitment to work with a "business as usual approach". It is possible to do a good job and keep performance levels up while pregnant. Believing this and projecting a positive attitude is essential. Maintaining good communication with your boss and giving adequate warning of any problems is a good idea. Employers appreciate knowing where they stand and appreciate a business-like approach.

Everyone has ups and downs at work and good and bad days. Just because you're pregnant doesn't mean you won't have the same. It is important to take these in your stride — there's no question of your commitment lessening because you have a run of morning sickness. If you keep it in perspective and carry on you'll find others at work will follow your lead.

2.   Women are the carers, men are the providers — therefore why are you still working?

You may find that many people change their view of you when you're pregnant. You are now a "mother to be", with the emphasis on mother. Mothers are caring people — pregnant women are vulnerable, moody, touchy, aren't they? It may be considered that you can no longer deal with demanding customers, handle negotiations with difficult clients, or anything else involving the harsh, stressful realities of working life. You would be better off at home getting ready to be a mother!

Of course, biologically women bear children and men do not, but the idea of women as nurturer and carer is so deeply engraved that it's hard to shake off. Even our language indicates this bias — children are "mothered"; we speak of the mothering instinct not the fathering instinct.

The only way to handle this blunting of your effectiveness is to tackle the misconception in a straightforward way. Actions speak louder than words. Continued good performance at work with little fuss will go a long way to getting people to drop these ideas about you and your pregnancy.

3. Now that you're pregnant you'll be looking for special treatment from all of us at work — you think you can have it all.

Many people feel that "you can't have it all" and some will even say it straight out to you. What they usually mean is they think straddling two roles is too difficult. It is a form of resentment and is often triggered by fear of an adverse effect on their workload or work performance.

It is up to you to show that you can do your work, that your brains are still intact and that pregnancy has not diminished your intellectual capacity in any way. Don't get annoyed or distressed with these reactions — simply deal with them.

REMEMBER — LET EVERYONE KNOW

- Your brain hasn't disappeared just because you are pregnant.
- You are committed to your job and you will be as flexible and hard working as always.
- You do concentrate on work while in work — you don't dream of your baby.

Amanda Willis, *a solicitor in a medium size company of solicitors, was quite apprehensive about being pregnant because so much of her work involved working with a senior woman partner who, although married, had never had children. She had always made it clear that she had put her career first and wanted no family. She had initially acted as a mentor for Amanda, thinking she was on the same path. Consequently, Amanda was a little apprehensive that her boss would think that she wanted it all and feel she lacked commitment to work. Amanda approached this dreaded task of telling her boss in the same way as preparing a legal brief. She was unemotional, kept to the facts and concentrated on the fact that she would be continuing her career and would be back at work after 14 weeks. She left no openings for personal exchanges. Her businesslike approach worked. Her misgivings were entirely misplaced! Her boss accepted her news and concentrated on the practicalities.*

Do you need to be assertive?

Assertiveness is a very important skill for any woman but now that your situation has changed with your pregnancy, it is even more important to develop it.

Assertiveness can be confused with aggression but is clearly different. You may already have your own ideas about assertiveness but the following are key elements of assertive behaviour.

KEY ELEMENTS OF ASSERTIVE BEHAVIOUR

- Having respect for yourself and for those around you.
- Not being dependent on others for approval and for your sense of worth.
- Being capable of asking clearly and directly for what you want.
- Being sensitive to the needs and feelings of those around you.
- Listening attentively to other people's views.
- Being open and straightforward with yourself and others and accepting responsibility for your actions and decisions.
- Realising that you have rights as do others — look at the list of rights later in the chapter.

Aggressive behaviour on the other hand involves being abusive and loud and not thinking of other people. It involves getting your own way by force, winning at any cost and in the extreme, hurting or humiliating other people.

SELF ESTEEM

You will see from the elements of assertive behaviour that an underlying core value is how you feel about yourself — your self esteem. Self esteem can be described as an inner picture of yourself encapsulating your strengths and weaknesses. This picture influences the way you relate to other people and what you can achieve.

As your body changes throughout pregnancy people's image of you as a working person changes. This changed perception can get in the way of effective communication and good working relations. It is all the more important at this time to retain your self esteem.

ASSERTIVE BEHAVIOUR WITH YOUR CO-WORKERS

Be confident and assertive in handling your pregnancy in work and be aware of positive and negative attributes and feelings in yourself and your co-workers. Be prepared to ask for any help you need from others without feeling your own self esteem is adversely affected.

Stand up for yourself and your right to work while pregnant with honesty and without aggression. Be prepared to accept responsibility for any problems it may cause and to deal with them effectively.

YOU HAVE RIGHTS TOO!

Before being assertive with others it's a good exercise to assert the fact that you have rights of your own. It's a basic precondition of assertive behaviour. There is a lot of talk nowadays about charters so why not work out your own charter of rights. The following points may get you started.

YOUR CHARTER OF RIGHTS AS A PREGNANT WORKING MOTHER

The right to be yourself.
As you move into your dual role of mother and worker remember to still think of yourself as an individual.

The right to ask for what you need.
As you juggle all your responsibilities and try to be as

efficient as always, despite your changing circumstances, remember you have a right to make requests of other people.

The right to be treated as an equal.
This is a fundamental right. However, as your pregnancy advances you may be a little less sure of yourself and may allow yourself to be treated as less capable or less intelligent than you are.

The right to have an opinion.
You always have the right to have an opinion and to keep it. You may find yourself under pressure when you're pregnant as many people, often older and not necessarily wiser, will try to convert you to their opinions. This is especially true when it comes to options for childbirth and childcare.

The right to express your feelings.
It's important to be able to identify how you feel at any point in time and to let others know how your feelings are affecting you.

The right to make a choice.
It's a clear right to be able to make choices and not have to justify them. Following on from making choices is the right to be able to change your mind.

The right to be wrong or to make mistakes.
When you make mistakes it is easy to become anxious and worried but everyone makes mistakes and you do have the right to be wrong.

Caroline Churchill, a sales representative, works very much to targets, and bonuses for reaching certain figures are important to her. Her sales manager pushed his sales team very hard and so far Caroline had coped with this slightly aggressive approach, albeit reluctantly. However, in the first three months of her pregnancy she was finding the going tough. She found all the extra trips, requests to visit yet

27

another client, very difficult, especially as she realised they weren't absolutely essential.

Caroline was faced with a dilemma: she needed to assert herself and establish some workable guidelines but now the situation was complicated by her pregnancy. If she chose to be assertive now it would look like she was using her pregnancy as an excuse for special treatment. This was certainly difficult and Caroline dreaded a confrontation. She raised the issue with a number of her female friends and talked it out female to female. It emerged that in many ways Caroline was the author of her own misery. Her behaviour in accepting unreasonable demands and not asserting simple rights, like going home on time, had placed her in this position.

The wisest thing said to her was "you can't change anyone else's behaviour, only your own". It was difficult but Caroline began to reassert her position, despite her pregnancy, she began to change her own behaviour, not her boss's!

Do you need to negotiate?

We all negotiate every day at home, in work, trying to reach agreement with other people. However, as a pregnant working woman and later as a working mother you will be negotiating many changes in work and at home, and the better you are able to negotiate the better deals you will get for yourself.

Negotiating is a process of give and take, of compromise. It is an activity you engage in when you are trying to get something you want from someone else. Successful negotiators know there must be a win-win outcome, i.e. something in it for both parties.

Although we are all negotiators, many of us, especially women, don't like to negotiate. They see it as stressful and confrontational. They don't want to fall out with people by trying to get their own way.

The key to successful negotiation is not to fall out with

the other side but to jointly come to an agreed solution. Professional negotiators are soft on people, "the other side", but hard on the issues being negotiated. For you, as a pregnant worker or returning-to-work mother, it can be difficult to be objective about negotiating maternity leave or alternative working arrangements. It is important not to take up a hard and fast position, but to concentrate instead on your interests and the other side's interests. This leaves room for negotiation.

Key to negotiation is the avoidance of open conflict or confrontation. The best negotiators do the unexpected, always look for openings to keep the discussion going. At the conclusion of every negotiation you want to have reached a mutually pleasing agreement in a friendly and open way. In negotiation the following are key factors for success.

KEY POINTS TO GET A WIN-WIN OUTCOME

1. Take time to **research and prepare well** before you begin your negotiation. Rehearse your arguments fully.
2. Whatever the other person's viewpoint don't react instantly, especially if you feel threatened, disappointed or hurt. **Stay cool and in control and focus on the outcome.** See this as just a stage of the negotiation to be gone through on your way to a successful conclusion.
3. Never, **never do battle and openly confront.** Whatever the reaction to you, don't argue. Try to understand the other person's position and don't act like a "gladiator" ready for battle.
4. If you keep your disposition positive and open and show that you are trying to understand the other's viewpoint you can then **suggest that you jointly try and seek a common answer** to this problem.
5. Be diligent in trying to **see the situation from the other's viewpoint** — you can't come up with a shared solution if you don't understand their needs.
6. **Don't expect miracles** — the person may still hold firm to their viewpoint despite your arguments. Don't push your viewpoint as it won't do you any good, concentrate

instead on finding a mutual solution combined of both viewpoints. Be creative in pushing forward to new solutions.

7. If you are having a difficult time and progressing nowhere show that neither side wins by giving in totally to the other. **Demonstrate that the best solution will be mutual.** It takes two to fight but only one to come up with a way forward.

8. **Know your own "walk away point"** or what you are willing to settle for at the end of the day. It may or may not be what you mutually asked for but make sure it's not less than you actually need. Never make instant decisions especially under pressure. Walk away if the going gets rough, and cool down.

FIVE TIPS FOR STAYING ON GOOD TERMS WITH EVERYONE IN WORK.

1. **Don't moan** about discomfort or draw attention to yourself, especially don't expect to be treated more favourably.

2. **Pull your weight.** Don't expect favours but if you do ask someone to cover for you when you go for a check-up, return the favour quickly. Be very diligent about saying thanks — don't take support for granted.

3. **Stay on top.** Use your 'to do' lists and plans to stay on top of your work load. If possible stay a little ahead of your work. Don't expect anyone at work to carry you — they'll be relieved by your attitude and actually be very supportive, as they realise that you are not going to dump on them.

4. **Talk about work loads with co-workers.** Be professional — discuss workloads and how you'll minimise the disruption effect of your pregnancy and maternity leave. Be realistic about the changes when you're going on maternity leave, you'll find people will appreciate being considered.

5. Be professional with your replacement if there is one. Make his or her job easy and you'll reduce disruption for your co-workers — this is a good long term strategy as you'll be coming back and you'll need them to fill you in and help you re-enter the work situation.

Judith Warren worked between two departments. Her work was quite tiring but because she was very fit and not at all sick she coped very well. The key to her success was her ability to negotiate with her companions at work. She traded jobs around and was always willing to pull her weight. It helped that many of the other staff were women who had families and so implicitly understood. However, her gift of negotiation came into its own at the end of her pregnancy when, although it was the Christmas rush, she was able to take maternity leave earlier than originally planned.

Can work routines be adapted to suit your pregnancy?

Many women contemplating pregnancy or in the early stages of pregnancy worry about being able to continue in their job with existing practice and routines.

For many, pregnancy causes only minor problems in work and they continue working productively right up to the end. For some, particularly if their job is very physical or involves working with chemicals or other dangerous substances, it is a different picture.

Since December 1994, special protection exists under legislation for employees who are pregnant. Employers must ensure now that your working conditions will not put your health, or that of your baby, at risk.

Remember if you can't do the same work as before due to pregnancy or recent birth or breastfeeding, it is unlawful for your employer to sack you.

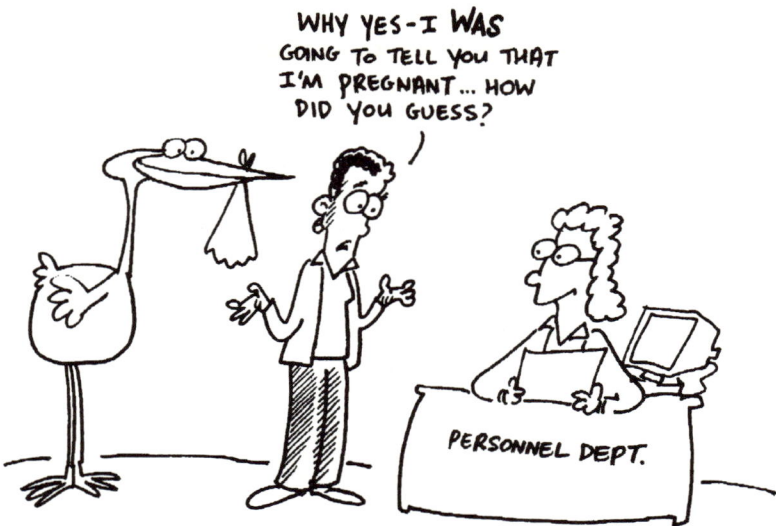

WHAT YOUR EMPLOYER MUST DO

There is now a legal responsibility on employers to assess risks to employees who are new or expectant mothers and to do what is reasonably practicable to control those risks.

There are a number of steps which your employer must carry out — briefly

1. A risk assessment of your work place.
2. If a significant risk is found do all that is reasonable to remove it or prevent your exposure to it.
3. Inform you of the risk and the action which has been taken.
4. If the risk remains, temporarily alter your working conditions or hours of work.
5. If the risk can't be avoided, offer you suitable alternative work.
6. If there is no suitable alternative work available — suspend you on full pay (or give you paid leave) for as long as necessary to avoid the risk.

The Maternity Alliance have excellent literature full of helpful information. Their address is in appendix 2.

WHAT YOU MUST DO

There are a number of things you must do in order to exercise your rights in this area of health and safety at work. You must tell your employer in writing about your condition and if he/she asks in writing for proof of your pregnancy show them your certificate of pregnancy from your doctor or midwife.

It is not essential but it is wise to discuss concerns you have about safety and your job with your doctor or midwife. You may be able to give your employer a letter from them which can be taken into account.

What are the hazards to pregnant women at work?

Hazards and risks of pregnant women are described under a number of headings.

- Physical agents
- Biological agents
- Chemical agents
- Working with VDUs

If you think any of these apply to you, you can ask your employer to go through the steps outlined earlier.

PHYSICAL AGENTS

These include regular exposure to shock, low frequency vibration or exercise movement. Lifting loads can also be a risk as hormonal changes can affect the ligaments and increase susceptibility to injury. Significant exposure to ionising radiation can be harmful to the foetus and so limits are placed on the external radiation to which pregnant women can be exposed.

Fatigue from standing or other physical work has long been associated with miscarriage, premature birth and low birth weight. Therefore, employers must ensure that hours and pacing of work are not excessive. If you require it seating must be available and rest breaks will also help reduce fatigue.

BIOLOGICAL AGENTS

Women working in laboratories or where they may come in contact with animals have to be careful as they may come into contact with organisms which cause damage to the foetus. If you work in this area consult your employer and your doctor or identify the risks clearly.

Teachers and other workers who have a lot of dealing with children should be alert for cases of rubella.

CHEMICAL AGENTS

For those women who work with hazardous chemical substances employers are required to assess the health risks to workers arising from such work and to try to prevent or control risks. Chemical agents are of particular concern if you work in the chemical industry, as a nurse, in the disposal of chemical or human waste, with pesticides or as a pharmacist.

WORKING WITH VDUs

Scientific evidence has not shown a link between working with VDUs and hazard to pregnancy. However, many pregnant women are still concerned, and because of this the Health and Safety Executive has consulted the National Radiological Protection Board (which in law must provide information and advice on all radiological matters to Government departments). They do not consider levels of ionising and non-ionising electromagnetic radiation from VDUs to pose a significant risk to health.

However, if you are concerned discuss it with your employer. It's wise when using a VDU to pay attention to your posture and to take breaks at frequent intervals.

NIGHT WORK

Although there is no immediately identifiable risk to pregnant women who work at night, if you have a problem and if you have a medical certificate stating that night work could affect your health and safety, your employer must take steps.

You should be offered suitable alternative day time work if any is available or you may get paid leave for as long as is necessary to protect your health.

Is there a need to revise your performance targets during pregnancy?

Any change in your ability to perform at work will be a concern to your boss and to the people who work with you.

When you announce your pregnancy to everyone at work move quickly to tackle their reactions especially if they perceive your pregnancy as meaning your performance will now drop off.

In the early stages of a pregnancy it's difficult to predict how things will go and to negotiate changed targets. It's best to assume that you will perform as usual and reach your normal targets. However, if circumstances change for whatever reason — you may be sick or very fatigued — then deal professionally with this and discuss it with your boss. It's not a sign of weakness to raise the problem and also to try to bring a solution.

It could be that you have negotiated some arrangements with co-workers to cover for you and you'll pay them back later. You could — if your job allowed — take work home, or change working hours, and in these circumstances keep up targets.

It's realistic to assume that in the final stages of your pregnancy you will be more tired and you will need to plan to accomplish less.

If you can predict that there will be a problem — be up front, perhaps you may need time off or sick leave. It's best to be honest — it's better appreciated than hiding and being found out when it's too late.

What about the final stages of pregnancy — the wind down?

As the date of the birth draws near you will begin to wind down. Usually women begin to feel quite tired and not able to work as hard. Some women sail on to the end but it's more usual to slow down — your sheer size demands it.

Make plans with your boss and your immediate co-workers about how your existing work will be covered while you are on maternity leave. You should make detailed arrangements if your work is being handled among your colleagues. You may want to identify clearly who is doing what and brief them on progress to date and expected results while you are out. You could introduce them to other people involved in the work both inside and outside your organisation.

If a temporary replacement is coming in — if at all possible and if your employer can afford it you should overlap for at least a week to successfully hand over.

Reassure those depending on you, like clients, customers, patients, parents. Tell them the work will be done in your absence and also let them know, if you can, who will be doing it. If you spend time ensuring a smooth transition there will be less confusion and it will reflect well on you.

FEELING ANXIOUS ABOUT LEAVING WORK

You may feel some anxiety about leaving the familiar world of work and taking so much time off. On the other hand you may be delighted with the new change in your life. Whatever you feel remember not to over enthuse or share these feelings in work. Your co-workers have to continue on in your absence and may be directly affected by it — so be careful not to rub it in.

Don't fall into the trap of reducing separation anxiety you may have by taking work home or promising to come in a few days after the birth.

Be firm, make your arrangements and go.

YOUR PREGNANCY PLAN

1ST TRIMESTER	2ND TRIMESTER	3RD TRIMESTER	BIRTH
1st week........	........12th week........	........26th week........	........39 week
The Tired & Sick Phase	*The Best Phase*	*The Large & Tired Phase*	

1st Trimester — The Tired & Sick Phase

- Read up on your legal rights about leave & benefits.
- If you are concerned about your health and safety inform yourself and then approach your employer.
- Visit your doctor or health clinic.
- Get literature about pregnancy and understand what will happen to your body.
- Start managing your time to retain productivity first
- Get a pregnancy survival pack together.
- Start your daily relaxation routine.

2nd Trimester — The Best Phase

- Decide which leave you are taking and which benefits apply to you.
- Mark your diary with dates for forms and letters to be sent.
- Schedule visits to doctor at start or end of day to reduce disruption in work.
- Inform your boss first.
- Inform your colleagues

3rd Trimester — The Large & Tired Phase

- Week 29. Earliest you can start maternity leave.
- Write to your employer 21 days before start of maternity leave and request maternity leave or extended maternity absence.
- Get your MAT B1 Form from your doctor.
- Start preparing for continuation of your work during maternity leave.

3 knowing your rights as a working pregnant woman

Being pregnant is a hugely important experience for any woman from the point of view of health, emotions, self esteem and re-adjustment. With all the turmoil this new event can cause to your life, it can be difficult to focus on the more mundane issues of leave and allowances. However, these issues are fundamental to the smooth management of your pregnancy and the sooner you get them sorted out the more time you have to concentrate on the less predictable aspects of your pregnancy.

You have legal rights as a pregnant woman at work. It is vital that you inform yourself of these and that you comply with any requirements asked of you. Employers vary in their knowledge of this area so don't depend on them to sort you out. This chapter will help you understand your rights and what you have to do to qualify. Use the chart at the end of the chapter as a guide. There are a number of more detailed publications available from organisations like The Maternity Alliance which will help you. They are listed in Appendix 2.

Can you be fired because you're pregnant?

No. The first and most important legal protection you have while pregnant at work is your protection against dismissal for any reason connected with your pregnancy, childbirth or maternity leave. It does not matter how long you have worked for your employer or how many hours a week you worked.

If you are dismissed and you believe that it is because of your pregnancy get advice from your trade union or advice bureau or a solicitor. If you intend to contest it you must put in your claim to the Industrial Tribunal within three months of dismissal.

Can you get time off for medical care or check ups or ante natal classes?

Yes, all pregnant women have the right to time off work for ante natal care. A great comfort is the fact that you are

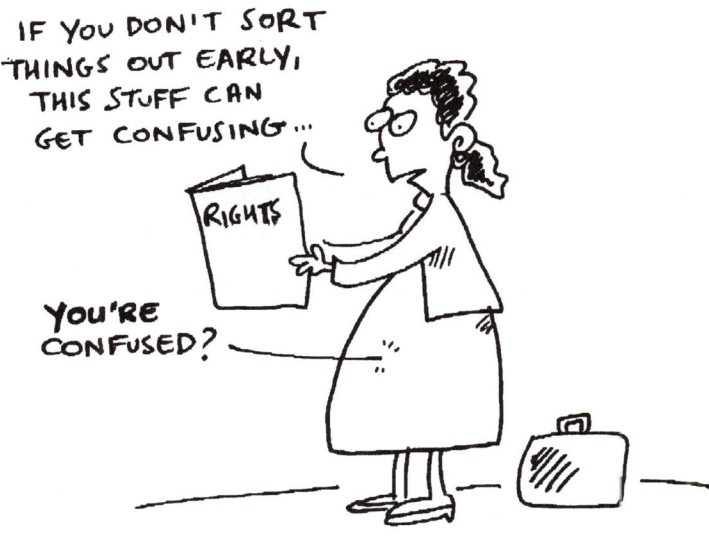

IF YOU DON'T SORT THINGS OUT EARLY, THIS STUFF CAN GET CONFUSING...

RIGHTS

YOU'RE CONFUSED?

entitled to be paid for such time off. You can take time off
not only for the actual appointment but also for the travel
time to and from the clinic or hospital.

It's important to be certain when dealing with
supervisors or co-workers that you are clear that all
pregnant women have this right, no matter what hours
they work, or how recently they commenced their job.

Ante natal care can include parent care and relaxation
classes. However, you may need a letter to show your
employer, from your GP, midwife or health worker, saying
that these classes are part of your ante natal care.

If the unfortunate happens and you are not allowed time
off or you are deducted pay you can make a claim to the
Industrial Tribunal within three months. Try to avoid this
if possible by educating your employers along the way.

Do you need to do anything to get this facility?

Yes, you should let your employers know when you need
time off and for how long you are likely to be absent. This
is also common courtesy and if handled well will go a long
way to creating a good impression with your boss and co-
workers. We discuss this in greater detail in Chapter 2.

After your first appointment your employer can ask to
see your appointment card and a certificate stating that
you are pregnant.

Are you entitled to any maternity leave?

There are two types of **maternity leave**: maternity leave
available to all pregnant women at work, and **extended
maternity absence** available to certain women fulfilling
certain criteria.

1. MATERNITY LEAVE

Are you entitled to any time off?

Yes. Any woman who is in work while she is pregnant is entitled to **14 weeks maternity leave**. This legal protection is quite clear. You are entitled to this leave if you are an employee, you do not need to have worked a certain number of hours a week or to have worked for the same employer for a certain length of time. If you have any problems with your employer there are a number of leaflets available which will explain this situation clearly. Useful contact names are given in Appendix 2.

Do you have to do anything to get your maternity leave?

Yes. You have to give notice in a special time frame and you need to tell them in writing. To qualify, simply write to your employer at least 21 days before you start your maternity leave. Tell him or her you are pregnant and give the expected delivery date of your baby. You must also state the date you intend to start your maternity leave. You only need to put this part in writing if your employer asks for it.

If your employer asks for it you have to enclose a copy of your maternity certificate. This is called form MAT B1. You will get this form from your GP or midwife when you are about six months pregnant.

If the unexpected happens and you cannot give 21 days notice — you could be in hospital with other things on your mind — you must write to your employer as soon as you can.

When can you start your maternity leave?

Let's consider the earliest possible date you can start —it's 11 weeks before EDD. From the earliest possible date on you can decide when you want to stop work. At the other extreme you can work right up until the week of childbirth.

An exception to this rule is if you have a pregnancy related illness or absence in the last six weeks of pregnancy. In this case your employer could start your maternity leave. However, if you are ill for only a short time your employer may agree to let you keep to your original plan for maternity leave dates. Consult the chart at the end of the chapter.

Do you lose your contractual rights while on maternity leave?

No, During your 14 weeks maternity leave all your contractual rights, like pension rights, holiday entitlements, your company car (if you're lucky enough to have one!) remain yours just as they would if you had been at work. Your monetary entitlements are dealt with in a later section.

What do you do about returning to work after your maternity leave?

This depends on when you intend to return to work. If you are going back at the end of your 14 week maternity leave you do not need to give any notice. However, in the section in Chapter 4 on returning to work there are some handy hints on this. When you go back to work, it will be to the same job.

If you want to return before the end of the 14 week period you must give your employers seven days notice in writing of the date you will be returning.

If, for whatever reason, you forget to give this notice and just turn up before anyone expects you, unfortunate things could happen. Your employer can send you away for seven days or until the end of your 14 week period, whichever is earlier.

Can you go back to work straight after you have the baby?

By law you are not allowed to work for two weeks after childbirth. If your baby is born late and you took a lot of maternity leave before your birth your maternity leave may have run out. In this case your maternity leave is extended by two weeks from the actual birth of your baby.

What happens if you're sick at the end of your 14 week maternity leave?

If this happens and you are unable to return to work you should be able to get sick leave from your employers. You are protected from unfair dismissal for an additional four weeks if you have given your employer a medical certificate before the end of your maternity leave.

EXTENDED MATERNITY ABSENCE

Some women qualify for **extended maternity absence** up to 29 weeks from the week of childbirth in addition to **maternity leave**.

Do you qualify for extended maternity absence?

- Women who have worked for the same employer for two years by the end of the 12th week before the due date, will qualify for this. Even if you have not got enough years to qualify at the start of your pregnancy you may have accumulated enough by the time you need to apply.
- You must work at least until the end of the 12th week before the baby is due.

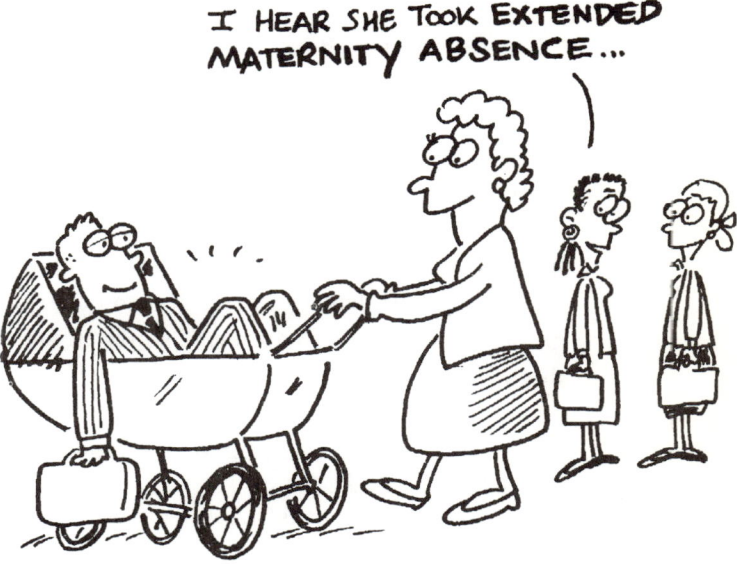

I HEAR SHE TOOK EXTENDED MATERNITY ABSENCE...

- Unfortunately, if you work in a company which employs five or fewer people you do not have a clear right to return after 29 weeks, even if you have worked the necessary hours. You do, of course, qualify for **maternity leave**.

Do you have to do anything to get extended maternity absence?

Yes. You follow the same steps as you would when applying for the 14 week maternity leave (see earlier section) but with one important additional point. This is worth considering carefully as it does bind you. You must write to your employer stating that it is your intention to return to work after the birth and you must do this at least 21 days before you start your 14 weeks maternity leave.

What time period does this maternity absence cover?

The extended maternity absence runs from the end of the 14 week leave period (to which every pregnant woman is entitled) until the end of the 29th week after your baby is born. It's important to remember to start counting the 29th week from the beginning of the week in which the baby is actually born. Look at the chart at the end of the chapter to clarify this.

What do you do about returning to work after your extended maternity absence?

At least three weeks before you plan to return, you must write to your employer and give notice of the exact date of your return — your NOTIFIED DATE OF RETURN.

However, your employer may take the initiative and write to you any time from eleven weeks after the start of your maternity leave, asking you to confirm that you are going back to work. **You must reply in writing within 14 days if you wish to return, or you will lose that right**.

CAN YOU DELAY YOUR RETURN BEYOND 29 WEEKS AFTER THE BIRTH?

No. In normal circumstances you must return to work. However, there are four exceptions.

1. If you are ill you can delay for up to four more weeks. You must send in a medical certificate and let your employer know before the intended return date.
2. Your employer may delay your return for up to four weeks. He/she must tell you the reason and give you a new date.
3. An interruption of work, e.g. a strike. In this instance you can delay your return until work starts up again. If the interruption stops you giving your notice of return date, you can delay your return for up to 28 days after the end of the interruption.
4. You and your employer may agree a delay. Obviously, this can cover any number of circumstances, and is subject to negotiation between you and your employer.

Are you entitled to pay and benefits?

There are two kinds of payment: **Statutory Maternity Pay (SMP)** and **Maternity Allowances**. You will receive one or other of these instead of your usual wages.

1. STATUTORY MATERNITY PAY (SMP)

If you're not sure about your entitlements to SMP ask for it anyway. Your employer will work it all out for you. You can get it even if you do not plan to go back to work and you don't have to repay it.

What is it?
- Weekly payment for women employed during pregnancy.

Who gets it?
- Women who have worked for the same employer for at least 26 weeks by the end of the 15th week before the baby is due.
- Are still in their job in this 15th week (holidays and sick leave don't affect this)

- Earn £61 per week or more on average (April '96).

How do you get it?

- Write to your employers at least three weeks before you stop work and ask for your SMP. Send a copy of your maternity certificate.

How much is it?

- You get 90% of your average pay for the first six weeks. (The average is calculated from your gross earnings in the eight weeks before the end of the 15 week before the baby is due). After that six weeks you get the basic rate of SMP which is £54.55 (Aug. '96) per week for up to 12 weeks. You won't get SMP for any week that you work.

When is it paid?

- SMP is paid for up to 18 weeks. It is your decision when you want to start your maternity pay period but week 11 before birth is the earliest you can start SMP. If you are ill in the last six weeks of your pregnancy, check whether you should be paid your statutory sick pay or SMP. Your employer should pay your SMP weekly or monthly, in the same way you are usually paid, after deductions for tax and National Insurance contributions.

MATERNITY ALLOWANCE

What is it?

- Weekly allowance for women who work before or during pregnancy but who don't get SMP. You can get Maternity Allowance if you are self-employed or if you give up work or changed jobs during your pregnancy.

Who gets it?

- Women who can't get SMP but who have worked and paid full National Insurance contributions for at least 26 of the 66 weeks before the week in which the baby is expected. If in doubt, claim and your Benefits Agency will assess you.

How do you get it?

- Get form MA1 from your ante natal clinic or Benefits Agency.
- Get your maternity certificate, form MAT B1 from your midwife or GP when you are about six months pregnant.
- Get a SMP1 form from your employer — it will give it to you if you do not qualify for SMP.
- Send in your MA1 to your Benefits Agency as soon as you can after you are 26 weeks pregnant. Send in your MAT B1 and SMP1 with it or later if necessary.
- If you have not paid 26 weeks National Insurance contributions by the 26th week of pregnancy, you can keep working into your pregnancy and send in the form when you have made the 26 National Insurance contributions.

How much is it?

- There are two rates. The lower rate of £47.35 per week will be paid to self-employed women and those women who are unemployed in the qualifying week (the 15th week before the expected week of childbirth). A higher rate of £54.55 per week will be paid to women who are employed in the qualifying week. There are no deductions for tax and National Insurance contributions

When is it paid?

- Maternity Allowance is paid for up to 18 weeks any time from 11 weeks before the expected week of childbirth.

What about weeks 18-29?

- If you have opted for extended maternity absence, remember that you may have no income after allowances finished after 18 weeks.

What are your health and safety rights?

If you are pregnant, have given birth within the last six months or are breastfeeding, your employer must make sure that the kind of work you do and your working conditions will not put your health or your baby's health at risk. To get full benefit from the new legal protection of your health and safety you must notify your employer in writing of your condition. This aspect is covered in great detail in chapter 2.

How can you negotiate your leave?

When deciding your leaving date try to be as flexible as possible. Remember the expected delivery date is not set in concrete and may be wrong. You may feel quite fit and active up until the very end. You might prefer to be in work rather than at home waiting .... and waiting.

Be generous with yourself when deciding the length of your maternity leave. A 14-16 week maternity leave gives you time to get to know all your baby's moods. Also an added bonus is that most babies have got a sleeping routine by then and may be sleeping through the night. This is a huge issue for working parents.

The most important consideration is your mental and physical health. You should not go back to work and take on the onerous task of being a working mother unless you are fully well.

Although your entitlement to maternity leave is protected by law, the exact start time and return date and the amount of contact you'll maintain with your work are open to negotiation with your boss. The way you handle this is as important as the way you announce your pregnancy.

- You should be as businesslike as possible, leave your emotions outside the door. Have your plan ready but be flexible and provide solutions to all your boss's problems.
- Don't be pressured into accepting something you feel unhappy about, like coming back earlier than your 14 weeks maternity leave.
- Be clear about how available you are going to be while on maternity leave and stick to it.

A GUIDE TO YOUR LEAVE AND BENEFITS

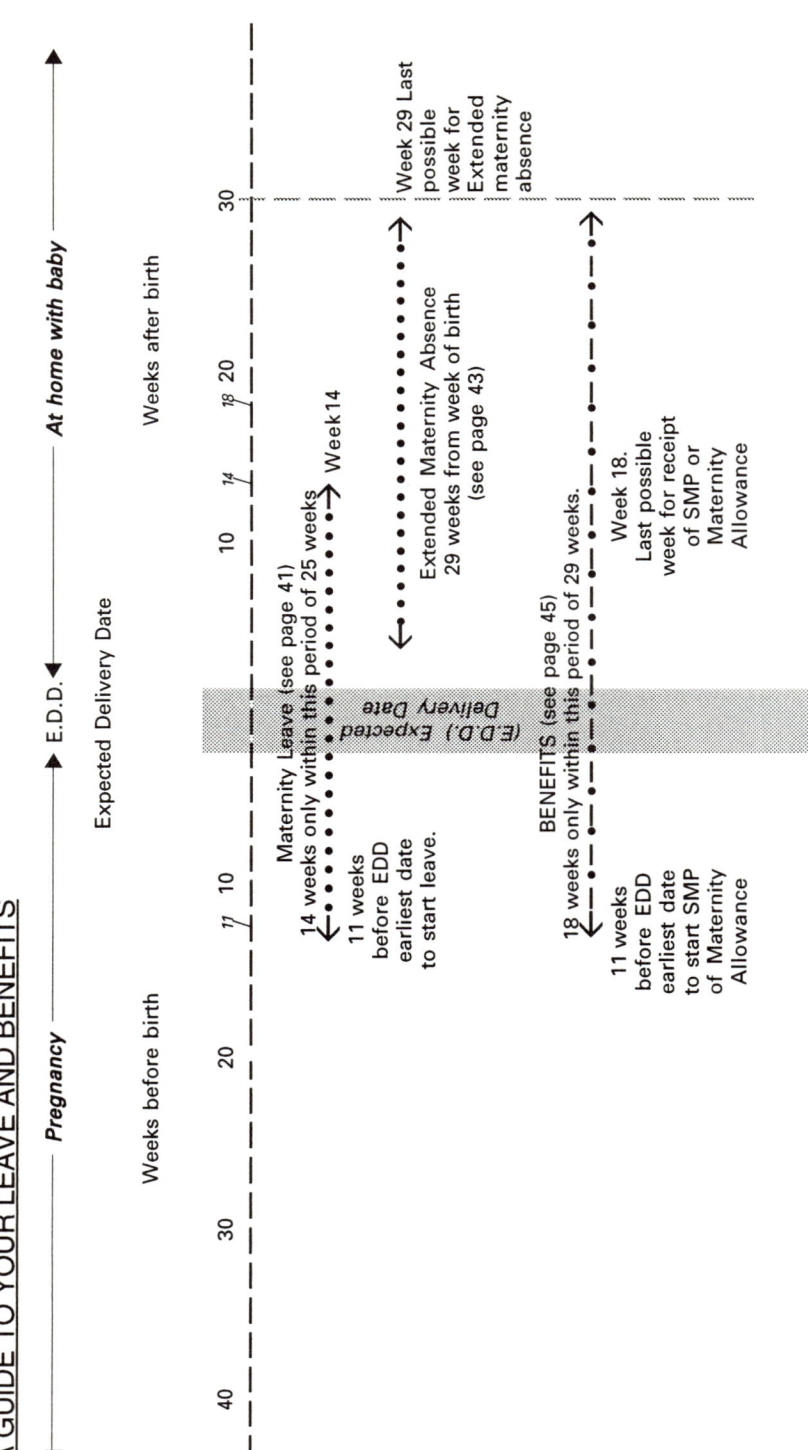

Pregnancy ◀────── ▶ E.D.D. ◀── At home with baby ──▶

Expected Delivery Date

Weeks before birth   Weeks after birth

40   30   20   11 10   (E.D.D.) Expected   10 14   18 20   30
                                              Delivery Date

Maternity Leave (see page 41)
14 weeks only within this period of 25 weeks
◀──▶ Week14

11 weeks
before EDD
earliest date
to start leave.

Extended Maternity Absence
29 weeks from week of birth
(see page 43)
◀────────────────────────────────────▶

Week 29 Last
possible
week for
Extended
maternity
absence

BENEFITS (see page 45)
18 weeks only within this period of 29 weeks.
◀──▶

11 weeks
before EDD
earliest date
to start SMP
of Maternity
Allowance

Week 18.
Last possible
week for receipt
of SMP or
Maternity
Allowance

50

4 returning to work after the baby

Deciding whether or not to go back to work after you've had your baby is a big decision and this chapter will help you. If you opt for part-time work the section on different types of alternative work arrangements will help you make an informed decision.

Once you've decided to return to work you'll find the **"EIGHT WEEK RETURN TO WORK PLAN"** useful and the **"FIRST DAY BACK SURVIVAL GUIDE"** will help you get through the first few weeks as a working mother.

Can you stay in touch during maternity leave?

Depending on your job and the level of responsibility you have, you may want to keep in touch with your work during your maternity leave.

You should have set out clearly how much contact you wished to have with your work during maternity leave, before you left work. The extent of contact will depend on the type of work you do and your seniority in the company. The size of the company is important, particularly if it is a small company and you have a senior management role.

For many women the role is simple, they leave for their 14 or 29 weeks, and the company hires a replacement to do their job for that period. Once you have trained in the replacement you can relax and disengage from the job for the period of your maternity leave. Shop assistants, bank clerks, receptionists and telesales people are examples of this kind of situation.

If you work in a large organisation and they issue newsletters, memos or notices to staff, arrange for these to be sent to you. You should ask to be kept informed of all job vacancies appropriate to your level.

If, however, your job is very much tied up with your particular skills and you have customers or clients who will only deal with you, the situation is much more complex. You could be in the legal profession and be intricately involved in a case or you could be a marketing executive dealing with one major client. In this instance, you will have to keep in touch with your office even if someone else is carrying out the day to day work.

If you are a very senior manager or chief executive, especially in a small organisation, you will not be able to disengage for the whole maternity leave. You must stay in contact as you have so much responsibility and it would be very difficult to replace you. It would take your replacement too long to "learn" the job, and you would be back just as they were getting on top of it.

If you are in this position you are very vulnerable as you may not get the break or peace and quiet you need at this important point in your life. The answer is to have a good plan ready.

Have your office install a fax at home and tell everyone to fax you and you'll phone them back. You're then available but your availability is under your own control. You won't have to answer some work query while you're in the middle of changing a nappy or breast feeding. You can phone back and answer all queries for the day when the baby is asleep.

Plan to be totally unavailable for five to six weeks after the birth. Act, and have everyone else act, as if you were on an extended holiday for the first six weeks, preferably on an island with no phone.

Have people report to you by fax every Friday, on the

week's work. This works best if you agree a 1-2 page report form before you leave. Always respond to the report and write your queries and instructions on it and fax back. If it comes through on Friday, you have until Monday to reply. That is easier at the weekend as your partner can allow you some free time to "think".

Louise Somerville headed up a small voluntary organisation and kept in constant touch during her maternity leave. This was done by her office sending faxes which she then answered as she had time. It worked well as the organisation was too small to have a new person step in for 14 weeks.

Lucia James, a cashier in a building society, did not need to keep in constant touch during her maternity leave. However, she was hoping to apply for a promotion, so she had all internal vacancies posted to her and actually went for an interview on her first week back at work, after maternity leave.

To go or not to go back to work?

Just as you have settled into a good routine with your baby, and your role as a mother and full-time homemaker, you have to think about giving it up and going back to work.

As the date of your return to work looms large on your horizon, don't underestimate the emotional upheaval associated with this time. Many mothers find this a time of intense soul-searching, when they question the whole idea of working, their career, their ideas of motherhood and the future of their marriage or partnership. Lack of sleep and genuine exhaustion can affect the judgement and equilibrium of anyone. Add sweeping hormone levels into the equation and you'll quickly see why this is a difficult time for most mothers.

For some mothers the choice is clear — they want to work

for financial, psychological, or other reasons. They never falter — well, perhaps for only a short while! Others cannot face leaving their child and either opt to stay at home or seek an alternative form of work involving less hours at work.

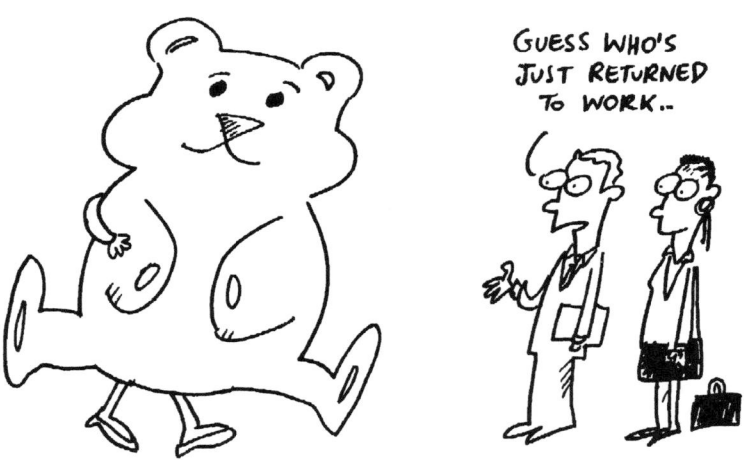

GUESS WHO'S JUST RETURNED To WORK...

Ultimately, it's down to personal choice whether to work or not. Whatever you choose is going to be right, if it feels right for you at the time. Beware all the experts with strong opinions you are going to uncover in these few weeks. People are very free with advice and can get cross if you argue with them. This is the time to remember your rights (listed page 25) and to be quietly assertive.

The best group of people to talk it over with, besides your partner, are women who have been through a similar situation. A note of caution: always remember when talking to people, copers always cope and whiners always whine, so temper their advice with a look at what kind of person they are.

When you make your decision, give it a while to see how comfortable you are with it. Don't make a rash decision about something as important as this, which will affect your life in a big way.

Read the section on alternative working arrangements and ponder the pros and cons of each.

Should you consider alternative work?

Flexibility is a much sought after commodity in a working mother's life, that, and sleep! The combination of your full-time job and your role of mother may leave you with little or no flexibility in your life.

You may want to explore alternative working arrangements which could reduce your time at work and give you more control over when and where you work You may feel completely overcome and think that life is no longer under your control.

Many women consider alternative working arrangements to give themselves more time with their children but also to retain a link with the world of "paid" work.

Consider carefully that leaving full-time work, and adopting another work arrangement, may not necessarily result in perfect harmony or lack of stress in your life. We'll explore the pros and cons of each alternative type later in this chapter.

IS THERE A DOWN SIDE TO ALTERNATIVE WORKING ARRANGEMENTS?

There is a down side in career terms to all alternative work practices. It usually means less money, less status, and possibly a slow down in your promotion. It can also mean considerable hostile reactions from co-workers who feel you are less serious about work and again having it all. The fact that you are being paid less for less time worked can be overlooked.

Some employers categorise professional working women, like solicitors, accountants, bankers and doctors, into two types: those who will not let their family affect their career and those who want both career and family in equal weight and so seek alternative work arrangements. A derogatory term applied to those who seem to want both is being "mummy tracked". If this happens to you it can mean getting less important or meaningful work and your career will be adversely affected. Watch for this and take action to assert your place.

HOW DO YOU DECIDE ON FULL OR ALTERNATIVE WORKING ARRANGEMENTS?

Carefully consider your finances before you begin this process. Your household budget must be able to sustain a sizeable reduction, remember also to add in the cost of any childcare arrangements you may need.

If you are really determined on getting an alternative work arrangement and your employer cannot help, you may have to have a contingency plan ready to find this kind of arrangement elsewhere.

In making your final decision weigh up the advantages against the disadvantages — neither are minor. You are making a decision which is fundamental to your mental and physical wellbeing. You should make a trade off and decide on the unique solution for you.

To help you decide, examine each of the following options and seek advice from organisations with specialist knowledge like *New Ways To Work In London — details in Appendix 2.*

What are the alternatives to full-time work?

There are four main arrangements

1. Part-time working/shorter hours

Deciding on a part-time arrangement is a bit like booking a holiday. You have to decide what you want, and what others important to you want. In effect find a solution that is likely to please all concerned and thereby influence the outcome. Then you have to live it to see if you have made the right choice.

The exact details can vary greatly from working 80% to 50% to 10% of a working week. You can work a couple of whole days or part days every week. This depends on what you work out with your boss.

Part-time working will have to be negotiated but consider that it is often low paid and has low status in companies. Certain industries can cope with this more easily than others e.g. the retail and grocery sectors.

In making your decision you should take into account the nature of your work; the rhythm of busy and slack periods over a week; the interaction of your job with everyone else around you.

In surveying your work and the work of those who work with you, take into consideration how flexible you will need to be. For example don't build up rigid start and finish times linked into baby care arrangements. Most jobs require some flexibility to cater for demands that you work overtime to fill orders, mind important clients, or supervise exams — any number of reasons which are hard to refuse.

A phenomenon called "elastic time" comes into play. You are expected to work 20 hours and get paid for 20 hours but for different reasons you are actually working 23-24 hours each week. Your pay is rigid but your work hours are elastic — in the end you may lose out.

Because of this phenomenon many part-timers find they work more hours than they originally anticipated. Be careful of this, keep a record and ask to be paid for these extra hours.

Gayle Adams worked in a small travel agency, and found that she only wanted to work 20 hours a week. She discussed it with her boss and negotiated an arrangement whereby she worked a 20 hour week most of the year but agreed to work longer during the three months when holiday bookings were at a peak.

2. Job share
This means two people sharing the same full-time job including pay and holidays. The actual division of time depends on you, the person you are sharing with and your employer. A variety of arrangements have been tried

including working week-on week-off; working two and a half days on and the same off; working morning on, afternoon off.

Obviously, in order to job share you have to find another person willing to share with you. You can do this by asking your co-workers or discussing it with your personnel department.

Care is required in choosing the person to job share with as both parties have to be sensitive to each other's needs and need to be careful to pull their weight. In choosing your "job sharer" consider your compatibility. It's vital that you get along and communicate well with each other. You should have complementary skills and training.

You may need to present a case to your employer, so think it out well. List all the positive aspects of two people doing one job. Presenting a written case will improve your chances. Lastly, remember your assertiveness and negotiation skills and use them.

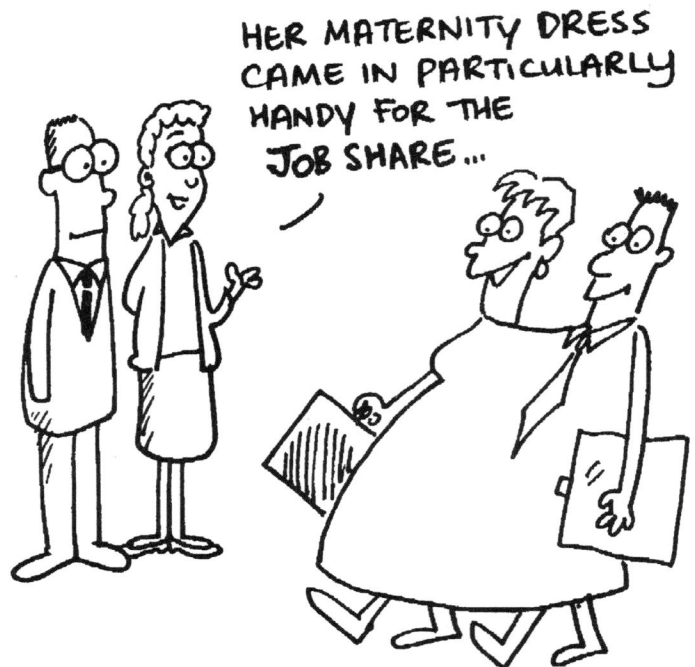

HER MATERNITY DRESS CAME IN PARTICULARLY HANDY FOR THE JOB SHARE...

Job sharing can often require more imagination from your employer than part-time arrangements. You have a bigger barrier to overcome. However, an immediate benefit is that you are less subject to the hazards of 'elastic time' as the job is being covered full-time between two people.

The down side can include the stresses associated with transition between two people, different working styles, capabilities and diligence. Conflict may occur over holidays, missed deadlines and rewards for tasks well done. If you have to cover for someone while they are absent due to personal sickness or sickness in a child, in any long term way, you can begin to feel put upon.

*Two women, **Martina Smythe and Jane Howley**, both worked in a large international service company. They both had two children and were finding the going a bit tough. However, they both enjoyed their work and wanted to keep a toe hold in the "working world". They got on well and were like-minded so they agreed to job share. They approached their boss together and negotiated a job share arrangement.*

3. Work from home
Flexibility in location rather than time is the key to this arrangement. It is an increasingly popular option particularly if your job involves the use of modern technology.

Working from home using a computer is ideal for computer programmers, editors, research analysts, writers, data processors and some types of organising secretaries.

It can also work if your job focuses on producing a body of work. Perhaps your boss will agree to you doing it at home and sending it to work via fax or modem.

Jobs involving a lot of telephone work can also be done from home, for example selling ads for newspapers, magazines, free sheets.

The most obvious benefits are not having to get "dressed for work" or having to waste time commuting. You can arrange your family life around your work and vice versa.

This is not a totally flexible arrangement. There are constraints associated with it. You cannot mind your child and work at the same time — if you think you can you may be setting yourself up for stress and disappointment. You need will-power in order to close the door on your child. As your child gets beyond the baby stage it may be necessary to have some form of childcare on call. In effect, you need to establish a boundary inside your home between work and family. Don't underestimate the difficulties, toddlers are ingenious at getting your attention and wasting work time.

As with the other alternative work arrangement you have to consider your status in the company and your long term prospects. In addition, be clear about your position in case you unknowingly become a freelance contractor and no longer an employee. You may be happy to accept a new arrangement like this but be clear about any change in entitlements.

Mandy Tenner worked on telesales for a newspaper, specialising in selling adverts for special features. There was no pressing reason why Mandy had to do this from an office. She had a special phoneline installed at home, billed to work, and did her work from there.

4. Flexible working hours

This system operates on a core working hours system which usually ranges from 10am to 4pm. Everyone is expected to be at work during these hours. You work up your quota of hours in the morning or evening around the core hours. This system can allow some flexibility in your morning hours. It is in effect a "shift" and not a reduction in hours — you have some flexibility without loss of pay or position.

Unless your company has a very hard nosed approach you should get a hearing when you propose a new arrangement. However, as with anything, the better prepared your case, the more assertive and clued into negotiation you are, the better you will succeed. This goes for all jobs at all levels.

WILL YOUR BOSS HAVE ANY PROBLEMS WITH ALTERNATIVE WORK?

There are a variety of arguments against alternative work arrangements by companies

"This has never happened in our company, field, or industry before."

Many companies don't want the risk of innovation but will readily copy a success from elsewhere. Find them examples of such successes and you will greatly strengthen your case.

"This will cost too much!"

This is an automatic response by some employers to any suggestions for change. This may frustrate you as you know they have no idea of the cost as they have never considered this system before. The real cost of replacing you and the lost cost of any training or experience you have acquired is often overlooked. Point out how valuable you are and how much it will cost to replace you if you leave.

"If we agree to this for you it will open a flood gate."

If we allow one employee to work part-time or job share, everyone will want the same privilege. This is often complete nonsense, not all women want children or want to work and have children. Help your employer to put your request into perspective.

"How can anyone working part-time focus on the job?"

An argument beloved of young, single bosses.

Your answer!

Your answer to all of these is to have a well prepared case ready, detailing other instances where alternative work arrangements have worked, any cost implications, numbers of other employees likely to go through the "floodgates" and any other convincing arguments you can think up. You may need help with this — consider organisations specialising in this and talk to other working women in similar circumstances. Learn from their mistakes.

How can you ease back into work?

Now that you've decided to go back, be it to full-time or any other arrangement, you need to start getting ready for the transition. You are going to leave your cocoon and "fly" back to work. In order to fly you'll have to do a lot of preparation so that you go back without any problems, and integrate the two parts of your life.

It's important to do this gradually and not just come to work one day and hope to take up where you left off. The following eight week EASE BACK PLAN should help.

YOUR EIGHT WEEK RETURN TO WORK PLAN

8 weeks before
- Organise your childcare arrangements — this is crucial as you cannot return to work if this is not sorted out.

4 weeks before
- Check your wardrobe and get your work clothes ready — take a good look at your wardrobe. It's a while since you were at work.
- You may need to buy some clothes to fit your new size or borrow some for a short while. If you wear a uniform it may need alterations.
- Pay particular attention to looking your best on your first day back.

2 weeks before

- Contact your work and get a brief update on what's happening. It also serves as a reminder that you will actually be reappearing. You might be a bit depressed if there was no place for you or that your temporary replacement was still there.

1 week before

- If you are having a childminder come into your home or bringing your baby to an outside childminder, start your baby this week. It will give you a week to practise and get used to leaving your baby. You can go over all your baby's special needs well in advance. It would be very unwise to leave all that to the morning you are going back to work.
- Stop in at your work for a short visit and show off your baby. While there, take home any paperwork, sales literature or materials to make sure you catch up before you come back.

Will you have back to work anxieties?

Yes, you will, everyone feels these, to be honest. It's common in the last days of maternity leave to feel like you're standing on a cliff looking at a thick fog. Be patient, the fog does clear. You do get on top. You may identify with one or more of the following common anxieties.

BACK TO WORK ANXIETIES

- **The first anxiety you will be feeling is about leaving your baby.** This anxiety will be eased if you have full confidence in your childminding arrangements. If you're comfortable about them, then you can focus on your adjustment to your dual role, rather than on your baby's.

- **You won't bond with your baby because you're working.** You may worry that you are returning to work before you have bonded with your baby. There is no evidence to suggest it happens but you may still feel this.

- **Your baby will be closer to your minder than you.** Most women have this feeling. You want your baby to like the minder but it's hard not to feel a little sense of loss as you see your baby with someone else. Once you recognise that you will have a touch of these feelings you can begin to deal with them and put them into perspective.

- **You will not be able to cope with both roles — worker and mother**. There is no doubt that the dual role is difficult but it is possible to do both. Chapter 5 will give you lots of advice on this.

- **You'll feel so guilty about leaving your baby that you'll be unable to work**. Be reassured — everyone suffers these guilty feelings. Working mothers can suffer intensely from guilt but so too can stay-at-home mothers but for totally different reasons. It's normal to feel guilty but you must keep it in perspective. Try to think of the positive side of your working, like you enjoy your job, you are contributing financially to your family budget. Then let the guilty feelings go, if you don't they can become destructive.

Will you get through the first day back?

- Your first day back is a huge event in your life. After all, you've been through the whole drama of childbirth, becoming a parent. You feel transformed and you're walking back into your old work place to meet everyone again. You'll be half expecting everyone to jump up and hug you. More likely people will say hello and go on as usual. Don't be disappointed or put off, it's just a usual day for

YOUR FIRST DAY BACK SURVIVAL GUIDE

- It's a good idea to start back to work on a Wednesday or Thursday, then your first week back will be shorter than normal, and you won't be tired at the end of it.
- Try to arrive at work half an hour early on your first day. You'll get ahead and stay ahead. Arrive looking professional and thereby make your entrance as a working woman coming back to work.
- Try to remain businesslike and keep talk about your baby and your childbirth experience to a minimum. Be as efficient and effective as possible on your first day back — you'll be pleased with yourself when you go home.
- Don't socialise at first, by planning lots of lunches or after work drinks. It will put you under too much pressure.
- Be prepared for changes in work, some months have passed and undoubtedly some things will be different. Don't be alarmed, you will get back on top very quickly.
- Check with your childminder quietly and don't make a fuss.
- Reassure your co-workers and your boss that you're back and focusing on your work. No better way than to throw yourself back into work to signal how glad you are to be there (whether you are or not). Once you've settled in, have lunch with your work friends and catch up on all the work news.

everyone in work.

- Remember all those misconceptions about you when you were pregnant, well, on your first day back, your boss and your co-workers are watching you for signs of being less serious about your work, obsessed with baby talk and likely to tell baby stories at tea break. **Remember the most important thing you are going to do today is to prove everyone wrong.** You are not really the larger waisted, sleep deprived, baby obsessed person they think. You are, in fact, an efficient, focused worker ready to get on with the next phase of your life.

You're back at work, now what?

Well, you've launched! You're back at work, you're now a working mother. Unfortunately, there is no clear cut map to tell you how to cope in these early weeks, but one thing is clear, organisation and advance planning will now be an integral part of your life.

You have made the leap of faith and you're a working mum. You'll find that you will be able to plan tomorrow and next week (maybe) but then things have to take care of themselves. Don't try to get in charge of everything, that won't happen, not until you retire!

The following sample work plan may help you in the first few weeks and months until you develop your own routine.

SAMPLE PLAN OF YOUR DAY

The night before

- Prepare your clothes and lay them out ready for the morning.
- Pack your requirements for work — briefcase, school notes, uniform accessories, whatever.

- Prepare baby bottles if you are taking your baby out to a crèche or minder.
- Prepare lunches if necessary.
- Get breakfast ready as far as possible and set the table.
- Write out your instructions for your childminder and keep them near your handbag.

In the morning

Get up earlier, as you will be amazed at the difference it makes. You'll have more time to get yourself and the baby ready. You'll be more in charge, and will leave for work in a calm state of mind.

After work

- Relax on the way home, before you have to gear up for the "evening shift" at home. Listen to relaxing music on a walkman or in your car.
- Eat a high protein snack an hour before you leave work so that you have enough energy for the evening.
- Leave your work worries at work and get ready for your home and family life. Your work problems will still be there in the morning.
- Concentrate on your baby and your family. This is the time of day when everyone is very tired and it can be quite a stressful time. Remember your baby can also be tired so take time to ease in.
- Talk things over with your baby minder. You can go over the baby's day and find out any problems. It also gives the baby time to adjust to your presence.
- Say good-bye to the minder. With a "good-bye ritual" your baby has the chance to say good-bye to the day and the minder and to switch to the evening.

In the evening

- Switch into evening mode. Change your clothes when you get home as this can help you change gears and relax.

- Prepare your evening meal in advance, possibly have a cook-in on the weekend and freeze the dishes.
- Focus on your child — do relaxing and enjoyable things with baby and enjoy your time with the baby.
- Save some time for yourself — even 10-15 minutes to recharge the batteries.
- Remember to try to go to bed early. You need lots of rest to keep up this pace; it's important not to become exhausted.
- Ask your partner for help in the evening.

Can you continue breastfeeding at work?

If you are breastfeeding during maternity leave you'll now be deciding whether or not to continue when you return to work. It's a difficult decision as if you do continue you'll find yourself the exception rather than the rule.

Don't underestimate the difficulties involved especially at this time when you will already be under enormous pressure.

To continue totally breastfeeding your baby is an option available to few women. It depends on having the baby minded close to work, in a work crèche, or if you're extremely lucky and work near home or near your minder's home.

If you decide that you want to, then some advance preparations will smooth the way. Introduce a bottle to your baby early on as a supplement to the breast. A good time is the 6-7pm feed each evening when your milk supply is low, because you're tired at the end of the day. This prepares your baby to accept both bottle and breast when you are back at work.

If this is not possible then a number of other options are available; you can easily feed morning and evening. Feeding during the day is more of a challenge. Some women express milk and store it, others use formula during the day.

Jackie, a Supervisor in a Customer Service Centre, had intended to continue breastfeeding when she returned to work and made all the advance plans. Unfortunately once back at work she realised that she was putting herself under enormous pressure. This was compounded when the effects of a major marketing promotion made their way through to her department and she had to work late a couple of days. She gave up and weaned her daughter completely. She felt that she had been a little idealistic in thinking she could continue but was glad that she had breastfed for almost three months.

5 how to make the most of your first year as a working mother

After the first few weeks back at work you'll wonder why you ever worried. Routines reassert themselves at work and you get into some kind of flexible routine at home. You're now a working mother, well and truly. Don't get cocky though, because about this time, the longer term considerations like exhaustion, stress and the danger of trying to be a "supermum" surface. This chapter will make you aware of common working mothers' traps and help you through them.

Are you doing too much?

If you ask any working mother what does she remember most from her first year back at work, she'll probably say **exhaustion**.

No amount of planning or time management will work if you are simply trying to do more than you have time to do. The easiest way to determine if you are taking on too much is to ask yourself, am I coping or do 1 feel overwhelmed? A good rule of thumb is if you feel overloaded then you are overloaded!

Sometimes you can deceive yourself and pretend that all is well, that this is what life is like for a new working mother. You carry on until you end up at the surgery every few weeks with colds, 'flu, and sore throats. Then the penny drops and you realise you are totally exhausted from trying to do too much.

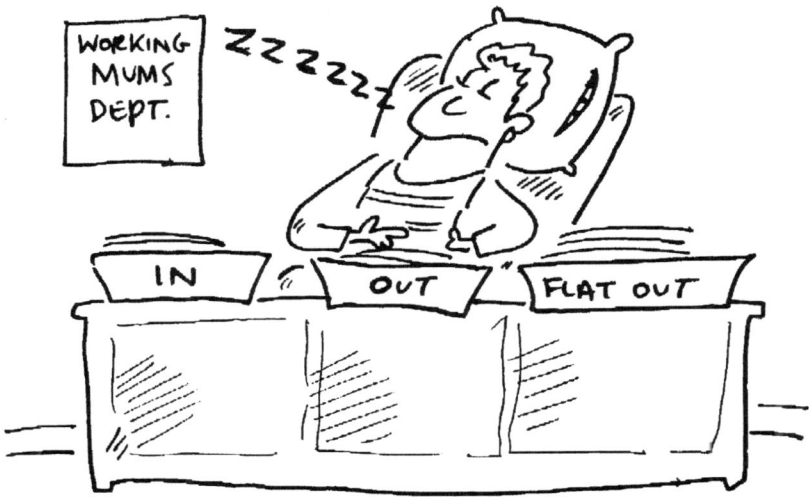

ARE YOU SUFFERING FROM SUPERMUM SYNDROME?

Trying to be a supermum is a huge trap many working mothers fall into. It's really carrying the myth of being a "superwoman", who can do everything to perfection, into the life of a working mother. The classic sign is the woman who, although she works full-time, organises a child, family and home, still seeks perfection in everything, as if she had only one of these roles.

Ask yourself these questions and if the answer comes up "yes" to a number of them, then you may be a supermum.

- Are you **exhausted** when you wake up, as well as when you go to bed?
- Are you **irritable**, prone to shouting, and crying?
- Are you feeling **unsupported** in all spheres of your life?

71

- Are you feeling **guilty** about not doing enough, not being good enough at everything?
- Are you feeling **angry**? Do you think you are self-sacrificing day in day out; week in, week out, and no one cares?

WHAT CREATES SUPERMUMS?

- **Protection of their family**

In order to protect their family from any loss due to their absence at work, women overcompensate. They try to protect their families emotionally, physically and socially by trying to do too much in too little time.

- **Guilt**

Natural maternal guilt about leaving your child can be fed and increased by setting very high standards for yourself and then not living up to your own unrealistic expectations of yourself.

HOW TO WEAN YOURSELF OFF THE SUPERMUM SYNDROME

- **Recognise the warning signs.**
  Accept that your feelings are valid and that they are telling you that you are expecting too much of yourself.
- **Reduce your expectations.**
  Ask yourself honestly whether your expectations of yourself are realistic or not. See the big picture; this is only a short period in your life, you won't always be in this position. Remind yourself that children grow up and become less dependent.
- **Be kind to yourself.**
  Allow yourself to feel bad, deprived and thoroughly fed up but with one proviso. Only do this for a limited time. Everyone is entitled to a "bad hair day" but it does you no good to wallow.

- **Slow down at home and at work.**
  You don't have to be number one in everything.
  Don't try to compete with "perfectionist
  housewives", who bake everything themselves,
  have homes designed to interior designer level,
  and wonderful high achieving children who
  attend four extracurricular activities after school
  every day. Don't compete because you have no
  chance, recognise that you're on a different path
  and do what you do best.
- **Seek help.**
  If you can talk to other women in your position
  who are coping, this can help put things into
  perspective and help you find the right balance.

Laurel Arnold was a classic supermum, but it took her until the end of her first year back at work to recognise that something was amiss. She found herself going to the doctor every three to four weeks in the winter, unable to shake off a sore throat or always on the verge of yet another bout of 'flu. Finally, the doctor asked her to tell him what she did on an average day, as a guide to her lifestyle. The doctor was genuinely amazed and told her so. Laurel had a rethink and a week off work to rest and recharge her batteries. Then she started looking at her lifestyle with a view to slowing down.

Why do you feel so stressed?

STRESS

Stress is often a by-product of a woman's choice to combine having a family and working full-time. In effect, stress is when you are no longer able to cope with what is going on around you in your life. You are overwhelmed and to a certain extent threatened.

The body's reaction to a threat is the "flight or fight" response. Adrenaline pumps around the body and the heart rate increases, pulse increases and the body is physiologically triggered to run away or stand and fight for one's life.

If you find yourself continually under threat the body remains constantly ready to fight and the accumulation of this can result in changed brain chemistry and high blood pressure, shallow breathing, less oxygen to the brain. All this results in you being crabby, unbearable and impossible to live with.

STRESS FOR WORKING MOTHERS

In the midst of the multiple demands being made on you by everyone around you it's important to pause and remember that if you don't look after yourself and you get sick you definitely can't look after anyone else.

Even when all is well in your life and you have a happy home, a healthy family, a job you enjoy, this period of your life as a working mother is probably the most stressful period in your whole life. You don't believe me! Well, consider some of the things which may want your attention: your child, children, partner, parents, school teachers, friends, children's friends, your boss, co-workers, house, repairmen, car, family pet . . . Sometimes all of these may want your attention all at once. Now you believe me, don't you?

Remember if you're not happy nobody's going to be happy! The first thing you must do is examine how many conflicting demands are being made on you and ask the question, how can I avoid taking on too much?

How can you avoid taking on too much?

You'll find the following will help you reassert yourself and help you cope.

1. Only do things that are really important.
Think before you take on any new commitment in your

home and family life. If you are going to devote some of your very precious free time to something new, outside your existing roles of mother and worker, it had better be very important. If it fails this "importance" test, don't take it on.

2. Get others to do things for you.

Get others to do things for you. This is a great idea and often overlooked by frantic working mothers, used to doing everything. Only do things you absolutely have to or you really want to. Don't fall into the trap of thinking you have to do everything at home for your family. Call on friends, family, or if you can afford it, pay someone else to do some jobs around the house. It is a mistake to think that you can do the same number of things that you did before you had the baby.

3. Concentrate on your priorities.

Your priorities will have changed now, and outside work you'll be trying to spend as much time with your child as possible. However, you'll also need time for yourself and your partner. In order to achieve these you have to prioritise.

Clarify for yourself what your priorities are on a daily and weekly basis. For example, if spending time as a family is a priority, you might want to make a rule of not going out weekday evenings, so that you can concentrate on your child and have an early night.

Don't over commit yourself, leave some empty space in your calendar so that you can take up the slack and really enjoy time with your child. Be clear about what things are important to you and do these first; then, if you run out of time only unimportant things are left undone.

Be firm about not responding to thoughtless or inappropriate demands made on your time, e.g. being asked to serve on voluntary committees, to entertain friends or have them to stay at your house during the working week. Usually people who have not been working mothers themselves are the most guilty of this thoughtlessness.

4. Be flexible

Don't impose unworkable deadlines or work loads on yourself. There are so many conflicting demands on you, both physically and emotionally, as a working mother that flexibility is the key to survival.

LEARN TO USE WORKING MOTHERS' MOST USEFUL WORD: "NO"!

This little word is often completely underused by working mothers. In their efforts to please everyone and to spread themselves in so many ways they forget how to say **"no"**.

Saying "no" gives you control. Saying "no" can free you from stress and pressure. It's time you started using it more frequently, especially when you begin to feel overwhelmed.

HOW TO SAY "NO" TO PEOPLE POSITIVELY!

- Listen very carefully to what you are being asked to do. Ask questions and fully understand what it will mean to you in terms of time and energy.
- Don't answer immediately — think.
- Decide if you are going to do it or not, and if you decide not to, say so immediately. Don't hesitate and say "I'll think about it", this gives the person the opportunity to persuade you. The non-committal answer gets you committed in the end.
- Don't be afraid of say "no". With so much on your plate you shouldn't worry about letting other people down. If you were looking for someone to do something for you, wouldn't you expect to have to ask a few people before you got a "yes".
- Soften your "no" with suggestions. Re-direct the person to someone else you know who would be willing to help. Offer to do some other, less time-consuming job for them.

Joanna Kane, a community worker, had huge difficulty saying "no" to people. Her whole life was becoming a drudge made up of work, housework and baby minding, sleep, and so on, in a never-ending cycle. She realised that she was staying late at work, arriving home late, exhausted, and she never seemed to get on top. She had to say to herself "no I'm not staying late — I've done my work, I'm going home".

By leaving on time she gained a whole extra hour each evening. Emboldened by this she also began to say "no" more often to other intrusions on her time and began to get slowly on top again.

Can you manage your time at home?

After a year or so working mothers become the best time managers in the world. Most working mums do a minimum of two things at once as it's the only way they can get everything done. Ask any working mum!

Time management was discussed in Chapter 1 and hints were offered for when you were pregnant at work. Let's now revisit these principles of wise use of time in relation to your time at home.

MAKE LISTS

Make a **master list** of all the big tasks that have to be done very week. Assign them to members of the household. Make sure that the task is the sole responsibility of that person or it'll all slip back onto you. Don't be tempted to do something which is left undone by someone else. If you do, it'll be yours again. Good tasks for this treatment are weekly shopping, putting out rubbish for collection, cleaning bathrooms, or cutting grass. If the rubbish piles up for two weeks then the message sinks home fast.

Make a **list of one-off jobs** to be done that week and mark them off as they are done.

KEEP A CALENDAR

Mark all household appointments on this and keep it in a visible place. This can greatly reduce confusion and double booking.

USE SHORT CUTS

Most household tasks lend themselves to short cuts. Stop being a perfectionist, remember the superwoman syndrome. Leave spring cleaning to spring, not every weekend. Only pick up toys once a day, preferably at night, and start afresh with clear surfaces and floors every morning.

CUT DOWN ON ENTERTAINING AT HOME

If you used to have lots of friends over for meals, carefully consider the time and energy involved in this before you start. Don't try and return favours-in-kind to people with no children who have all the time in the world to cook lavishly. Go eat their food and return the favour some other way.

If you do entertain at home, buy ready prepared food. If you feel guilty, hide the wrappings and say nothing. Another suggestion is to ask everyone to bring a different course. Concentrate on the good company and forget about the niceties of the menu.

USE THE APPLE PIE APPROACH

You no longer have the time to devote large blocks of time to chores. Instead chip away at them by doing a little every so often and eventually that wallpaper will be stripped or those plants will make it into the ground. This is detailed in Chapter 1.

REMEMBER THE PARETO PRINCIPLE

At home as well as in work, 80% of your output will come from 20% of your effort, so prioritise what you want to do.

If you're undertaking home improvements concentrate your efforts on making life easier for yourself e.g. a bigger, more organised kitchen might be more useful to a harassed mum than a new front drive. This is detailed in Chapter 1.

LEARN TO DO TWO THINGS AT ONCE

This is a vital skill in getting things done, so that you can make time to relax or go to bed early and get that much needed sleep. Some examples are, read your child a story when your evening meal is cooking, or tidy up or cook while talking on the phone. You'll find your own examples very quickly once you start thinking like this.

Kathy Horgan, a journalist, felt that she ought to keep on with the kind of life she had before she had her daughter, Amy, and so she continued to have dinner parties each weekend. Because she worked different hours each week, she was a great list maker. She made lists of everything and bought things well in advance. She cooked in advance and used her freezer. She also used convenience food and concentrated instead on the wine and the company. She felt that keeping this aspect of her life was important enough to put the extra organisational effort into retaining it.

Are there good times for working couples?

Many people believe quality time does not exist. There is a feeling that it's something invented by a working mother to make herself feel less guilty.

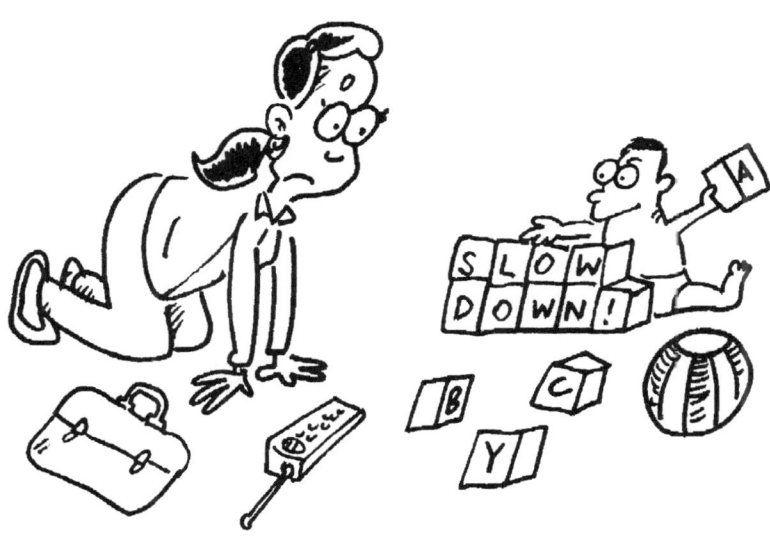

Not true, quality time does exist but it has to be created, and then carefully minded. Anyone who has sat on a park bench having a picnic on Sunday morning knows the difference between talking about nature with your children and snatching a few words with them in ad-breaks during children's television.

Quality time is when you and your child are together and aware of each other. You are enjoying the same thing, at the same time. You are out for a drive together or reading together or just quietly sitting together looking at people going by. There is no reason why working mothers can't have this just as well as anyone else!

Unless you plan to have quality time each week there is a danger that it won't happen. What is important, is simply being together without distraction.

QUALITY TIME AS A COUPLE

Do you feel that your life as a couple could go on the endangered species list? If you do, it's time you found a regular baby-sitter and went out every Saturday night. It really doesn't matter where you go as long as it's together and it's a child free zone. Sometimes the pressure of trying to go to entertainment which starts before 8pm or 9pm can make you wonder why you bothered. If you feel like this, just go for a walk, a drink, a drive, or go and visit some friends. Spending time with people who have no children can be good for you, as it stops you both becoming "baby bores".

BAD TIMES: WEEKDAY EVENINGS — THE POISON HOUR

In the chapter on returning to work we planned an average work day routine to minimise stress and fatigue. At this stage of being back at work for a few months, you'll probably find that the most stressful hour in the whole day is around 6 o'clock, when everyone comes in from work.

It's a well recognised cause of stress and has been called many things (mostly impolite), the best one to describe working women's true feelings for it is the **poison hour**.

Picture the scene: everyone comes home tired, blood sugar levels are low and there is a lot of crabbiness about. The television is on, new bills have arrived in the hall, there's no time to read letters, the phone rings, a meal must be made, children want your time, your partner wants to tell you about his day and you want to tell him about yours — is calling it the poison hour an understatement?

This is the time to slip into a well thought out plan and take hold of the evening before it rolls you over.

9 WAYS TO SURVIVE THE WORK DAY EVENING

1. **Change your clothes**. Get out of your working clothes, no matter how casual they are. It symbolises the fact that you're home and ready to relax.

2. **Banish interruptions**. Don't answer the phone or if possible use an answering machine. It's no accident people are phoning at this time; they are targeting you. Remember your priorities and don't march to someone else's timetable. Increasingly, telesales people operate at this time, don't get caught.

3. **Have rules about your children's time.** Try to have their time free in the evening, e.g. if your baby is being minded at home, try to have him/her already fed, or at least the food prepared before you come in.

4. **Try not to cook from scratch**. Pre-cook food on the weekends, use your freezer, buy in one or two pre-cooked meals and have the occasional take-out. Get a fast food meal now and then, use it as a treat for your children.

5. **Involve your children in chores**. Don't try to do everything in the kitchen on your own, while your child is elsewhere. Have him in his chair or buggy beside you. When he gets older let him help.

6. **Do something enjoyable after your meal**. Try to avoid slumping in front of the television like a family of couch potatoes. Well, try not to do it every night! Go for a quick walk, play in the garden, do a jigsaw, unpack the toy box and sit on the floor playing.

7. **Have a fun bed time routine for your child**. Children love routines so make the going to bed one fun. Start with a play bath with loads of toys, progress to reading a story, playing a game with their favourite stuffed animals and end by listening to a children's tape or watching a light show on the ceiling. You'll work your own routine out together but you'll notice how relaxing for both of you it is if you remove all the hassle from the procedure.

8. **Have some adult time**. Remember you're in this together with your partner, so do remember each other. Now you can quietly share your news about the day and plan the rest of the week.

9. **Go to bed as early as possible**. Sleep is your best friend, without it you can't keep up this hectic schedule, so don't be tempted to stay up late. Always remember you could be up at 4 am, dealing with teething.

GOOD TIMES: WEEKENDS — AN OASIS OF CALM OR AN ENDLESS LIST OF CHORES

There is a tendency to leave all chores to the weekend, e.g. going to the dry cleaners, going grocery shopping, gardening, vacuuming and other delightful housework duties.

There is a danger that you can spend all weekend doing your household duties! Some working women feel that to compensate for having been off "enjoying" themselves at work during the week, they must do "womanly" things at the weekend. You know the kind of household things women are supposed to do!

This is nonsense. Weekends should have a lot of fun built into them. Do all your tasks but be vigilant about planning in some family fun.

appendix 1

Childcare options

Having good childcare and being happy with it is crucial to a successful return to work, particularly from the emotional point of view. Leaving your baby every morning is hard enough, but if you're not confident that your baby is being looked after, you will not be able to concentrate on work and may end up feeling stressed.

Often women hesitate about making their arrangements as they don't want to face having to "hand their child over". They put off the search for a minder as long as possible. They want someone else to come along with an instant solution. Unfortunately, this rarely happens and bad decisions can be made as time runs out and the fear grows that some arrangement must be made, no matter what!

It is never too soon to start looking and finding out names and addresses. You don't have to go and see people too early but if you know your file on possible childcare options is growing it does keep you calm. Ask everybody for names and addresses, you'll find that the informal grapevine can be wonderful.

FOLLOW YOUR INSTINCTS

Deciding which form of childcare you want is a very personal choice and depends on emotional as well as physical factors. You might find yourself unable to leave your baby in a large crèche and feel you want one-to-one attention. If this is the case follow your instinct and stick it out until you find an arrangement which is going to make you happy. No one arrangement is better than another but feeling confident about it is vital.

Despite the bewildering array of jargon associated with this area your options break down into three main areas: having your baby minded in your home, someone else's home or in a crèche or day nursery.

Before considering your options, it's a good idea to be familiar with the law and the protection it offers you and your child. It strengthens your hand when interviewing people, as you know what the required standards are.

Childcare and the law

Since 1991, legislation entitled the Children's Act has regulated this area. Briefly, this Act

- regulates the provision of day care
- promotes good practice
- points out the duties of local authorities regarding day care.

Local authorities must keep a register of organisations or individual childminders who provide full-time, part-time or out of school care to one or more children under the age of eight. *Anyone who offers day care for payment, for a period greater than two hours a day, must register.* There are some exceptions, including: a relative caring for your child, foster parents, or someone who cares for your child in your home or who works for you or another set of parents and who cares for the child in one of your homes.

Before being registered the person will be assessed to see if they are suitable to look after children under eight. The assessment covers many angles including qualifications, physical and mental health, and any previous criminal activity involving children. The actual building may also be checked to see if certain standards are met.

You should check with your local authority register if you have any queries, but also because they may be an excellent source of information about what's available.

Option 1
Childcare in your home

MINDER

Having someone mind your child in your home causes the least disruption to your child and yourself. You can go to and from work without disturbing your child. This is particularly useful in the morning if you have to go to work early as you can leave the baby asleep. Another good point is that your minder does the travelling rather than you and your child. These invaluable people are called nannies or minders, for ease we'll use the term minder.

The minder will look after your child in your home and should do additional tasks associated with the child like food preparation, and clothes washing. Light housework is a point for negotiation between you and her. A note of caution, don't push your luck! Reliable, honest, and loyal people are hard to come by, but a dirty floor can be cleaned anytime.

LIVE-IN MINDER

If your minder lives in, you have a far greater degree of flexibility and this option can be very suitable for women whose jobs involve long or unpredictable working hours. However, as always, there is a trade off, as you lose your privacy and some space in your home. It's worth carefully considering this option before having someone enter your life in this significant way.

Having a minder in your home can be the most costly option but it does offer you greater freedom and greatly reduces your physical workload.

Some reservations exist about using a minder, chief of which is your total dependence on this one person. If she gets sick you can be badly stuck. Amazingly, minders coming to people's homes are among the most dedicated and hard working people and rarely seem to get sick. Yes, yes, exceptions do exist! But they only prove the rule. However it's no harm to have a back up plan ready for those emergencies when the minder can't come.

MOTHER'S HELP

Some women use a mother's help if they are working from home or only leaving the house to work for a short number of hours. They are usually young and inexperienced and so should work under your supervision, providing a backup to you.

FAMILY MEMBERS

Family members can often turn out to be the best minders but it's wise to take care to have clear cut arrangements worked out in advance. You should be clear about start and finish times for the working day and be businesslike about what you are going to pay and when. It's better to pay something as it keeps it on a business level.

When you have a family member you have the big plus of a familiar face for your child and someone you can trust. However, as with everything, there are some negatives. Emotions can run high in families, and relations, especially older ones, have their own way of "rearing children" and may not want to listen to your way of doing things. Unless handled well by you, this can cause trouble. If you are not very calm and clear about this and something goes wrong, you could lose, not just a child minder, but a favourite aunt or even worse fall out with your mother or your mother in law!

Option 2
Childminder in her own home

Another option is a childminder who will look after your child in her own home. She will have to be registered. This option provides the child with a home environment and the experience of being looked after in a normal home. The minder might be minding other children or may have some of her own so that your child can have company as he/she grows up. The disadvantages include having to bring your child out of the house in cold weather or early in the morning.

HOW TO FIND A MINDER

Get a shortlist

Start looking as early as you can. You can advertise in local newspapers or stick adverts on notice boards in local shops or supermarkets. Never give your address, just a phone number as this allows you to keep anonymity. You can check with any registers or agencies and put the word out among friends, relatives and neighbours. A person who comes personally recommended by someone you trust is a big bonus.

When someone gets in touch with you, perhaps in reply to your ad, try to get an overall idea of the person.

This whole process is wearing enough without wasting time meeting people who are totally unsuitable. Think about it carefully before you ask someone to come and meet you. If you have any doubts after your initial phone conversation don't continue — trust your instincts.

First of all, give some details of what you require as this may weed out some people straight away. Note down the basics like name, address, age, prior experience, phone number and any references.

These details will help you eliminate some people who are unsuitable because they live too far away, are too young or lack sufficient experience. After this process you should have your shortlist ready for a personal meeting or "interview".

MEET THEM IN PERSON — THE INTERVIEW!

You should prepare for your interview, but remember to be kind to yourself as this may be the first time you've interviewed someone. Aim to interview only one or two in a

day. Don't do what a friend of mine did and have eight
people come in on the one day, one after the other. She
was hiding in the garden by the end, unable to open the
door and face another stranger. Get a note book so that
you can note any major points or contact names and
numbers. It's very easy to get confused between people,
especially when you see a lot in a short space of time.

Carry out your interviews in two stages. First interview
the person without the child or children present, so that
you can concentrate and really listen to the person. Then
have the children brought in and observe the person
interacting with them.

If you're looking for a minder in your own home have
them come to you. If on the other hand the minder is
minding in her own house it's best to carry out this stage
while visiting them. If the house is unsuitable then you
can check that out first before introducing your child into
the process.

Once you're down to one or two people, at the second
stage, introduce the minder to your child or children. You
can then see how they get on together. This will be
particularly important to you.

You should discover if the minder has any training, or
previous experience. Most important it is worth discussing
what you would like to happen during the day. Will she
take the child for walks, what food she will use, and if she
shares your views about bringing up children. You must
know this so that you can be clear in your directions at a
later stage to the childminder.

Ask open questions like, "how do you feel about..?" "tell
me what you think about...?". When you have asked the
questions, wait and listen, you may be nervous and wish
to fill the silences — don't. Let the person speak for
themselves and listen carefully. Sometimes what is not
said can be just as revealing.

You may find yourself selling the job rather than
interviewing. Don't be too hard on yourself, as you are to a
large extent trying to start a very important relationship
with someone and you do have to sell yourself a little.

CHECKLIST FOR INTERVIEWING POTENTIAL MINDER

For any minder

- AGE — maturity.
- PREVIOUS EXPERIENCE — references.
- TRAINING — has she had relevant training?
- NEARNESS TO YOUR HOME OR WORK — potential problems with transport.
- CHILDREN OF THEIR OWN — company for your child.
- DEPENDANTS — do they have anyone totally dependent on them? Could this mean they could have a conflict of interest and let you down?
- PERSONALITY — is the minder child-centred or more interested in housework?
- OPENNESS — will they do what you want or do they have rigid views on childminding?
- CHARGE — if they appear to be very cheap, beware — they may be doing other jobs, even at night, to make ends meet and may be too tired to mind your baby.
- DOES SHE SMOKE? — a definite no.
- HOLIDAYS — will she take holidays at the same time as you?

In case of minder in her own home

- HOW MANY OTHER CHILDREN WILL BE THERE?
- WHAT AGES ARE THEY?
- IS SHE REGISTERED?
- CAN YOU TALK TO OTHER PARENTS USING HER?
- IS THE HOUSE SAFE FOR CHILDREN?
- WHAT FOOD WILL SHE GIVE YOUR CHILD — YOURS OR HERS?

OPTION 3
Crèche or day nursery

Many women prefer to use a crèche or day nursery rather than place their child under the care of one person. Nurseries look after a range of ages, and provide all day care in a registered and controlled environment. You must use a different approach when choosing a nursery, as you are not now focusing on one person exclusively, but on the whole package — owner of nursery, staff, numbers of children, their ages, and most important, the staff-child ratio.

FINDING A NURSERY

You may be one of the lucky ones, where you or your partner has a work place nursery. Certainly, if you are, check that out first. There are also private, voluntary or local authority nurseries. Check phone books, local papers, and ask friends, neighbours and relations. It does reassuring if you can get a personal recommendation.

As many of the better ones have long waiting lists it does no harm to put your name down early in your maternity leave, even if you leave your investigation of the place until later, when you're physically able for it.

WHAT TO LOOK FOR IN A NURSERY!

You're looking for a well run and friendly place, where your child will be comfortable and well looked after. So you have to examine two aspects, the staff and the way everything is organised. Firstly make sure the nursery is registered and that it is complying with the terms of the Children's Act regarding premises and staff.

Visit the place and observe closely what's happening. Is there an air of competence, how many children are there and what are they doing? A vital question is are there enough staff for the number of children? You'll find the recommended ratios for a nursery below.

AGE	STAFF TO CHILDREN RATIO
Under 2 years	1-4
2-3	1-4
3-5	1-8
5-8	1-8

Ask about the training of all staff, not just the person in overall charge. Check daily routines to ensure your child will get enough sleep, food and exercise, particularly outdoor exercise. If you've finally decided on a nursery, drop in unexpectedly to see how things look when you're not expected. Do talk to other parents, they are a wonderful source of inside information.

A friend of mine had some misgivings about a particular crèche, although it was difficult to focus on any one problem other than her child seemed quite overactive on weekday evenings. Eventually she began to turn up at 2pm in the afternoon, much earlier than expected. She found the crèche organiser asleep as well as most of the babies. It didn't take long to figure that all the youngest children were being left in their cots for long stretches of the day. No wonder they were slightly manic each evening.

A final word — remember you are an "employer" now

You are now employing someone to look after your child, be they in your home, or in theirs, or even in a day nursery. You may not be used to this role and it may take some adjustments in your mental attitude and behaviour. This is very important, because your ability to go to work depends on the success of this arrangement. Don't let this dependence over-influence you. As always, follow your gut instinct. If you're unhappy about something, investigate further and mention it up front.

Be clear about your and your baby's needs, and give clear instructions to the minder. In the early days, write down all your points for the minder. After a while both of you will grow beyond this.

As you are jointly managing the baby it's important to know everything that happened when you were away from him or her. At the hand over time, exchange information on what the baby ate and drank, and numbers and kinds of nappies. That way you won't miss picking up signs of constipation or underfeeding or approaching illnesses.

This might all seem daunting as you begin but in a short time, when you've established a routine, it will all slip into place as if you've always been a working mother.

One last point. If you employ a minder, you are legally obliged to keep a proper payroll record and to pay her income tax and national insurance contributions. This can take a lot of time and be quite complicated. You will master it but you might want to use a service like Nannytax — contact numbers in Appendix 2.

appendix 2

List of useful contacts & addresses

Pregnancy

HEALTH PROMOTION INFORMATION CENTRE
at Health Education Authority, Hamilton House,
Mabledon Place, London, WC1H 9TX.
Tel: 0171 383 3833
Health Promotion Information Centre houses the national
collection of health promotion materials. Useful publications
in areas of pregnancy, parenting and child health and
women's health.

To order contact HEA Customer Services, Marston Book
Services, PO BOX 269, Abingdon, OXON OX14 4YN
Tel: 01235 46 55 65

HEALTH & SAFETY EXECUTIVE
HSE Information Centre, Broad Lane, Sheffield S3 7HQ.
Tel: 0541 54 55 00
The Health and Safety Executive enforces the Health and
Safety at Work Act 1974 and advises on occupational health
and safety. Useful book — A GUIDE FOR EMPLOYERS; NEW
AND EXPECTANT MOTHERS AT WORK.

THE MATERNITY ALLIANCE
45 Beech Street, London EC2P 2LX.
Advice Tel: 0171 588 8582
Office Tel: 0171 588 8583

A national charity which aims to improve the care, health, education and social support given to parents, before conception, during pregnancy, childbirth and in the first year of their child's life. Very valuable information on rights at work and benefits.

THE NATIONAL CHILDBIRTH TRUST
Alexandra House, Oldham Terrace, Acton, London W3 6NH.
Tel: 0181 992 8637
A national charity which offers information and support in pregnancy, childbirth and early parenthood. It gives individual help and support and answers the most commonly asked questions about pregnancy and parenting.

Working mothers

WRN - THE WOMEN RETURNERS' NETWORK
100 Park Village East, London NW1 3SR
Tel: 0171 468 2290/1/2
The Women Returners' Network provides a free nationwide information service covering all aspects of returning to education, training or employment, newsletters and meetings. They provide excellent resource lists on grants for further education, sources of information, setting up your own business, flexible working options, childcare options and social security for women returners.

HOME - RUN
Active Information, Cribau Mill, Llanvair Discoed, Chepstow Gwent, NP6 6RD
Tel: 01291 641 222
Home-run is a newsletter published ten times a year and available by subscription only. It offers useful information and contacts in a wide range of areas, to people working from home.

NEW WAYS TO WORK
309 Upper Street, London N1 2TY
Tel: 0171 226 4026

New Ways to Work is the leading organisation (a charity) in the UK advising on more flexible ways of working. They publish very useful books, booklets, and a quarterly newsletter. Contact them if you are thinking about a different approach to your work.

OWN BASE - WORKING FROM HOME
68 First Avenue, Bush Hill Park, Enfield EN1 1BN
Tel: 01440 820348

Membership is open to everyone working from home and is a voluntary organisation run by its members, for its members. They promise that you should never be alone with your problems.

EQUAL OPPORTUNITY COMMISSION
Overseas House, Quay Street, Manchester M3 3HN
Tel: 0161 833 9244

The Equal Opportunity Commission is a public body set up by Parliament. It works to remove unlawful discrimination on grounds of sex, and to promote equal opportunities for women and men. Its staff provide expert advice, verbal and written, to the thousands of people who want help with a problem involving sex discrimination.

NATIONAL EXTENSION COLLEGE
18 Brooklands Avenue, Cambridge, CB2 2HN
Tel: 01223 316 644

Excellent reference materials and correspondence courses, reasonably priced, on lots of useful topics like career and business skills, personal and people skills and good support of GSCEs, A Levels and degree and professional studies.

Support groups for mothers

La Leche League (GB)
BM 3424
London WC1N 3XX
Tel: 0171 242 1278
La Leche League is a charitable organisation which aims to provide information, encouragement and support — primarily through personal help — to every woman who wishes to breastfeed her baby.

M.A.M.A. - THE MEET-A-MUM-ASSOCIATION
14 Willis Road, Croydon, Surrey, CR0 2XX
Tel: 0181 665 0357
It is a nationwide organisation which aims at providing a network of care to help all mothers and mothers-to-be. More than 70 groups nationwide which help you if you are a new mother feeling isolated or lonely. Especially useful for anyone suffering from post natal illness.

NATIONAL WOMEN'S REGISTER N.E.W.
3A Vulcan House, Vulcan Road North, Norwich NR6 6AQ.
Tel: 01603 406 767
N.W.R. aims to welcome all women. They offer the opportunity to take part in informal discussions exploring a wide range of topics, both serious and light-hearted. Most members belong to local groups which plan their own programmes. If you're lonely and would like to talk to other women contact them.

One parent families

GINGER BREAD
London Office:
16-17 Clerkenwell Close, London EC1R 0AA
Tel: 0171 336 8183

Northern Ireland Office:
169 University Street, Belfast, BT7 1HR
Tel: 01232 231 417
A charity run by lone parents for lone parents. It has a network of self-help groups, providing support and helping people to develop new skills and confidence. Excellent publications including "Free to Work" a comprehensive guide to childcare for England and Wales.

THE NATIONAL COUNCIL FOR ONE PARENT FAMILIES
255 Kentish Town Road, London NW5 2LX
Tel: 0171 267 1361
It is a registered charity working for the prosperity and independence of lone parents. Useful publications free to lone parents.

Childcare

CRY-SIS — SUPPORT GROUP
B.M. Cry-sis, London WC1N 3XX
Helpline available 8am - 11pm every day
0171 404 5011
Cry-sis is a voluntary self-help organisation run by parents who have experienced the problem of a crying, sleepless, or demanding baby or young child. They have a network of volunteers who run a telephone helpline. If you have this problem this could be a valuable help.

PARENTS AT WORK
Fifth Floor, 45, Beech Street, Barbican,
London EC2Y 8AD.
Tel: 0171 628 3565
Parents at work is a national charity committed to the welfare of children of working parents. Membership entitles you to a copy of "Working Parents Handbook". It provides a comprehensive guide to all forms of childcare options, information on employment rights at work for parents. There are support groups, bi-monthly bulletins and publications.

EMPLOYERS FOR CHILDCARE (EFC)
Cowley House, Little College Street, London SW1P 3XS
Tel: 0171 976 7374
Employers for Childcare is a forum of some of the United Kingdom's major employers who have first hand experience of trying to implement childcare and family-friendly policies. They are working for a national policy and strategy on childcare to meet needs of flexible and mobile workforce and to alow parents to balance and fulfil both family and workplace responsibilities.

If you want more information in this area get their literature, it might interest your employer.

NANNYTAX
PO BOX 988, Brighton, BN2 1BY
Tel: 0273 626 256
Nannytax is a payroll service, based on a simple annual subscription fee. They keep a payroll record and pay relevant income tax and national insurance contributions to the proper authorities on both your and your nanny's behalf.

DAYCARE TRUST
6 Wild Court, London WC2B 4AU
Tel: 0171 405 5617
They offer advice and information to parents and providers of childcare as well as to employers and professionals interested in childcare issues. They produce a range of publications, briefing sheets and a magazine called "Childcare Now".